Gorgeous Wedding Hairstyles

A STEP-BY-STEP GUIDE TO 34 STUNNING STYLES

by

Eric Mayost

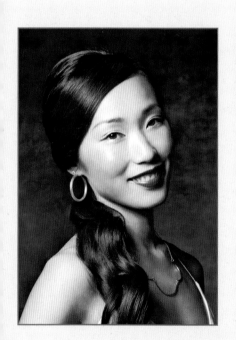

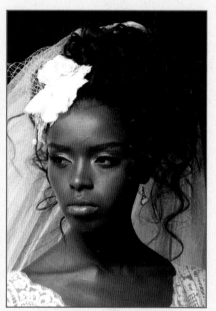

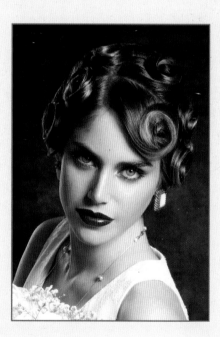

STERLING

New York

STERLING
New York

An Imprint of Sterling Publishing
387 Park Avenue South
New York, NY 10016

Created by Penn Publishing Ltd.
www.penn.co.il

Design and layout by Ariane Rybski
Photography by Roee Fainburg and iStockphoto
Edited by Shoshana Brickman
Styling by Louise Bracha
Makeup by Sigal Asraf

ISBN 978-1-4027-8589-4

Distributed in Canada by Sterling Publishing
c/o Canadian Manda Group, 165 Dufferin Street
Toronto, Ontario, Canada M6K 3H6
Distributed in the United Kingdom by GMC Distribution Services
Castle Place, 166 High Street, Lewes, East Sussex, England BN7 1XU
Distributed in Australia by Capricorn Link (Australia) Pty. Ltd.
P.O. Box 704, Windsor, NSW 2756, Australia

For information about custom editions, special sales, and premium and corporate purchases, please contact Sterling Special Sales at 800-805-5489 or specialsales@sterlingpublishing.com.

Manufactured in China

10 9 8 7 6 5 4 3 2 1

www.sterlingpublishing.com

Contents

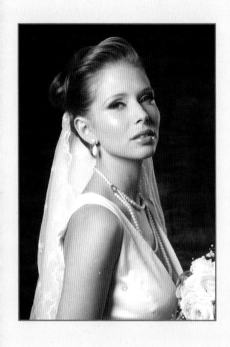

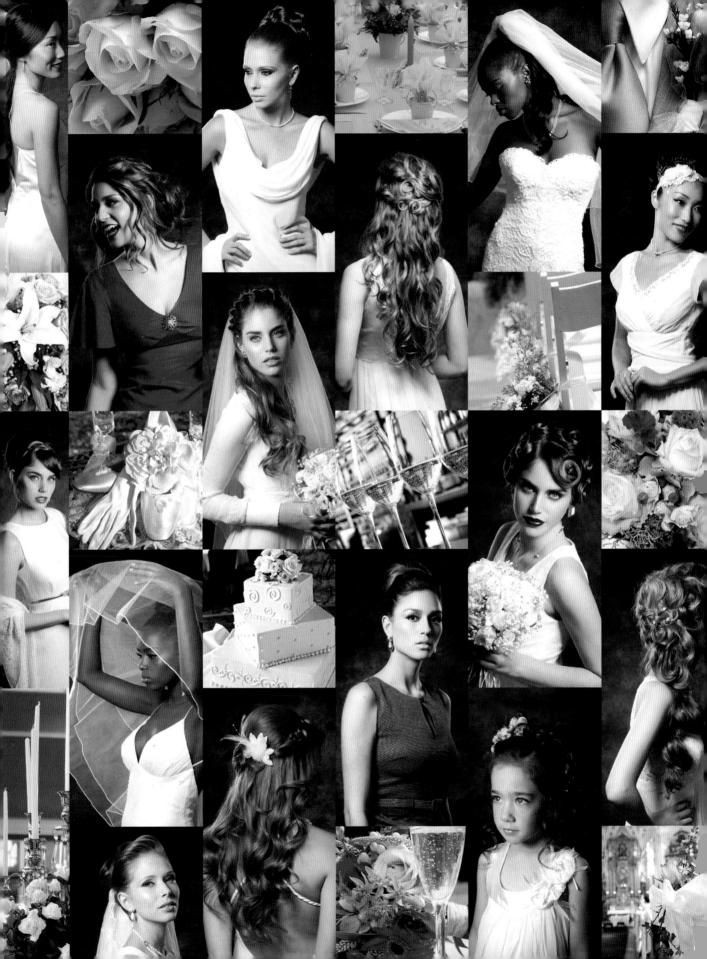

Introduction

Having the right hairstyle is part of having the perfect wedding day and **Gorgeous Wedding Hairstyles** is just the right book to help you make sure this happens. It features more than 30 beautiful hairstyles that were designed with brides in mind. There's something for brides with every type of hair and style. There are also several designs for other members of the bridal party. Every hairstyle includes easy-to-follow instructions and plenty of step-by-step photographs.

Invite a good friend over and try out a few hairstyles before selecting the one you want for your Big Day. Not only will you save money by styling your own hair, but you'll also enjoy the thrill of knowing that you were directly involved in your own fabulous hairstyle!

When your wedding day arrives, you won't need to adapt your schedule to fit in an appointment with a hairstylist. With **Gorgeous Wedding Hairstyles** in hand, you'll be able to have your hair done when you want it, in the comfort of your own home, and without paying high salon prices.

Once your wedding is just a beautiful memory, this book will still be on your bookshelf, ready to help you create beautiful hairstyles for other occasions. That's a good thing considering all the romantic anniversaries you have to anticipate!

ABOUT THE AUTHOR

Eric Mayost has been styling hair since he was nineteen years old. In addition to hairstyling, he studied art and graphic design. Eric has worked with some of the world's leading hairstylists and has participated in cover shoots for some of the world's leading fashion magazines. Eric has managed his own hair salon since 2002 and is the author of the bestseller **Spectacular Hair**. He has carved a career for himself by creating glamorous hairstyles that stars love, and enjoying staying at the forefront of hairstyling fashion. In this book, Eric shares the valuable tools, techniques, and experience he has acquired with his readers.

Essential Supplies

BLOW DRYER
Use this to dry freshly washed hair before styling it. In some cases, you may also need a blow dryer for the styling process.

BOBBY PINS
These small pins are used to secure the hair close to the head.

CURLING IRON AND HOT ROLLERS
Both of these are used to curl hair. Curling irons are easy to travel with, and great for using when you want to control the direction of the curl. Hot rollers are convenient when curling the entire head of hair. A double-barrel curling iron can be used to make waves in hair.

DIFFUSER
Use this to add volume and accentuate hair that has been curled.

ELASTIC BANDS
Use these to secure ponytails and braids. Choose ones that are gentle on the hair and don't rip it. Neutral colors are best, since they may be visible in some hairstyles.

HAIR ACCESSORIES AND FLOWERS
Many of the hairstyles in this book feature accessories to enhance the finished look. Of course, flowers are always a great accessory for bridal hairstyles.

HAIR CLIPS
These are used to hold sections of hair during the styling process. Metallic clips with sharp teeth are used to create sharp waves.

HAIR EXTENSIONS
Natural or synthetic hair additions are integrated into hairstyles to add volume and length. Hair extensions may be long or short, straight or curly, braided or left loose. Good quality hair extensions can be reused many times.

HAIR WRAP
This variety of hair extension comes wrapped in a sheer net. It usually looks like a removable bun and is used to increase volume.

HAIRNETS
These can be used to wrap hair (or hair extensions) to create a base in a hairstyle.

HOLDING SPRAY
Mist this onto the finished hairstyle to ensure that it lasts a long time. In some cases, you'll also want to mist the hair during the styling process in order to hold a particular shape. I usually recommend spraying from a distance of about 8 inches so that the holding spray is evenly dispersed on the surface of the hair. When spraying a specific area, you may want to move in a bit closer.

MOLDING WAX
Applying this to the hair helps sculpt it and achieve a strong hold. A little wax goes a long way, so apply a bit to the palm of your hand and then rub it into the hair.

SPONGES
These can be integrated into hairstyles to add structure and volume. To avoid having them visible in the final hairstyle, choose ones that are similar in color to the hair.

TAIL COMB
Also called rattail combs, these combs have teeth at one end and a fine point at the other. Use the teeth for backcombing hair and the fine point for making parts.

VEILS
Bridal veils come in many styles and designs. The ones used in these hairstyles are attached to a simple white hair comb which makes them easy to insert and remove.

WAVE IRON
This is used to crimp hair into waves.

WIDE-TOOTH COMB
Use this to separate locks of hair.

The Bridal Veil

There are so many different styles of bridal veils to choose from! Make sure the veil you select complements the design and fabric of your dress – and your hairstyle.

I recommend selecting a veil that has a small comb attached to it. Inserting this comb into your styled hair secures the veil in place. Try on the veil with your hairstyle before your wedding day and consider how you want to position it – do you want to insert the comb above or below the focal point of the hairstyle? Once you have decided where the comb will be inserted, create a base to support the comb by backcombing the hair in that part of the hairstyle.

INSERTING AND REMOVING

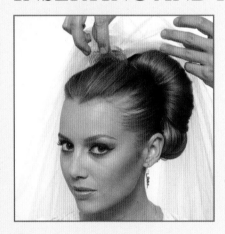

1

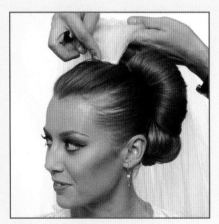

2

1. Select a veil that is attached to a metal or plastic comb. Make sure the veil complements the design and fabric of your dress, and suits your hairstyle.

2. Decide where you want to insert the comb before you start styling the hair. During the styling process, build up a base to support the comb by backcombing the hair in that spot.

3. Style the hair as desired. When the hairstyle is finished, gently insert the comb. Make sure you push the comb in straight so that it can be removed by pulling it out in the opposite direction. Also, make sure to push in the comb deep enough so that it is entirely concealed by the hair.

4. When you are ready to remove the veil, gently pull out the comb in the opposite direction.

Inserting and removing the comb is simple, and shouldn't have any impact on your hairstyle. Practice before your wedding day to make sure you get it right.

Glamorous TWIST

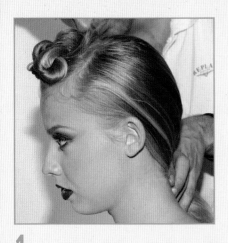

1. Wash and blow dry the hair. Mark a triangular part at the brow and gather the hair at the front of the head in a clip.

2. Gather the rest of the hair in a low ponytail at the back of the head, slightly to the side.

3. Affix three hairnets to a pin and secure them to the ponytail. Make sure you select hairnets that match the color of the hair.

4. Divide the hair into three sections. Backcomb one section from the roots to increase volume.

1

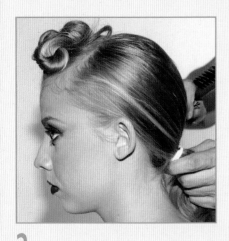

2

Evoke the romance of a 1920s film with this classic design. Feminine and elegant, it features a smooth wave at the front and an indulgently wrapped back.

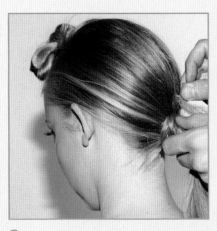

3

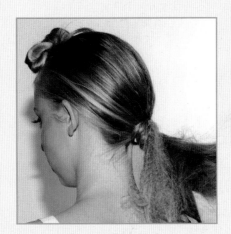

4

1

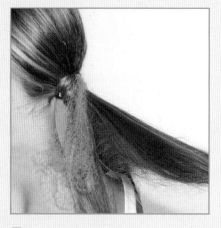

5

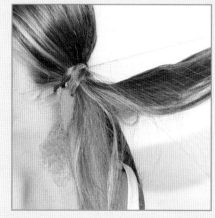

6

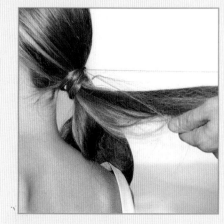

7

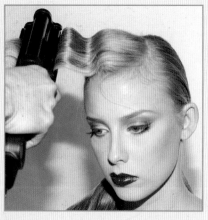

8

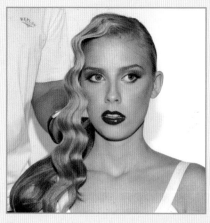

9

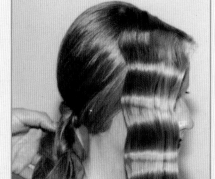

10

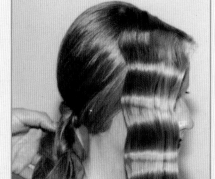

11

5. Gently brush the top layer of this section and mist with holding spray.

6. Wrap this section of hair with a hairnet.

7. Repeat the same procedure with the other two sections of hair.

8. Remove the hair clip from the hair at the front of the head. Mist the hair with holding spray and style with a wave iron to create waves.

9. Make sure the waves reach the ends of the hair and then let the hair cool for about 5 minutes.

10. Return to the back of the head and make a basic braid using the three groups of hair wrapped in the hairnets.

11. Make sure you don't make the braid too tight because you want to preserve the volume. Secure the end of the braid with an elastic band.

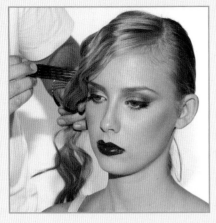

12

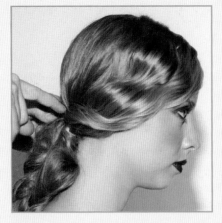

13

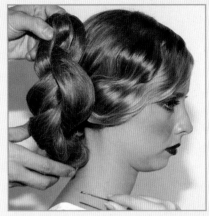

14

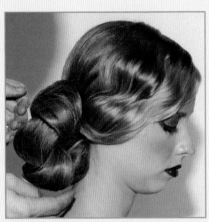

15

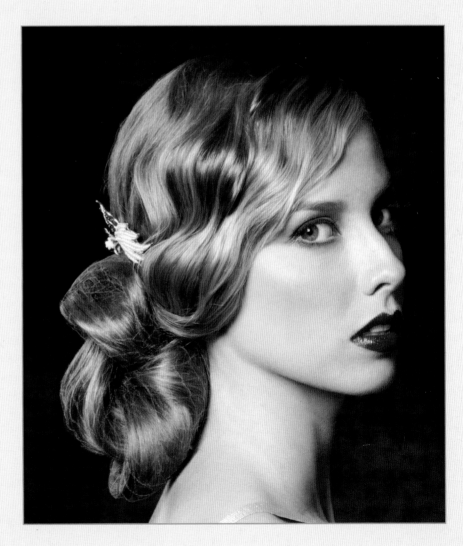

12. Gently draw the wavy hair from the front of the head towards the braid. Make sure you don't damage the waves.

13. Secure this hair at the top of the braid with bobby pins.

14. Sweep the braid upwards to leave the neck bare and position as desired at the back of the head.

15. Secure the braid with bobby pins and mist with holding spray.

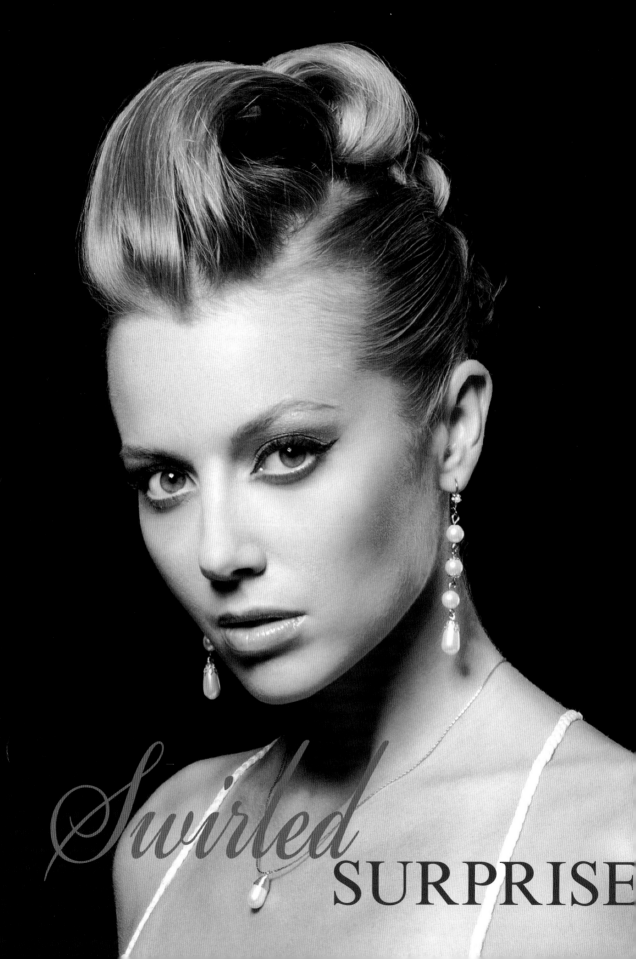

Swirled SURPRISE

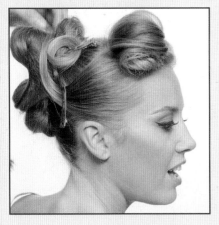

12

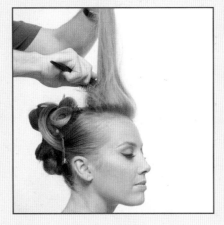

13

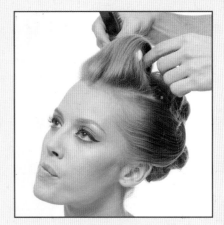

14

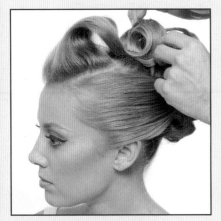

15

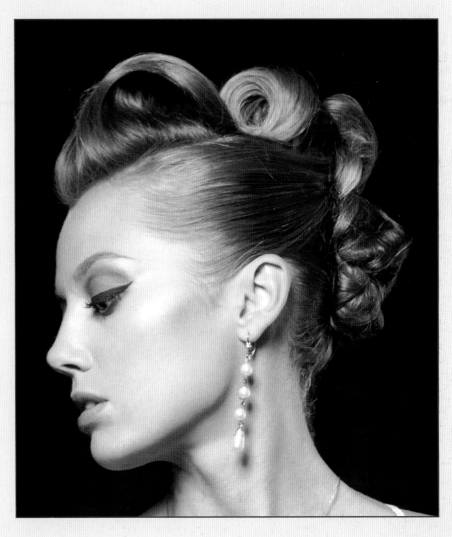

12. Shape these sections of hair as you like and secure to the scalp with bobby pins. Continue to shape the ends of the hair along the sides of the wrapped sections of hair and secure them with bobby pins.

13. Backcomb the bangs close to the roots.

14. Roll the hair backwards to allow for volume and then secure with bobby pins.

15. Roll the ends of the hair into curls that blend in with the sections of hair that you've already sculpted. Secure with bobby pins and mist with holding spray.

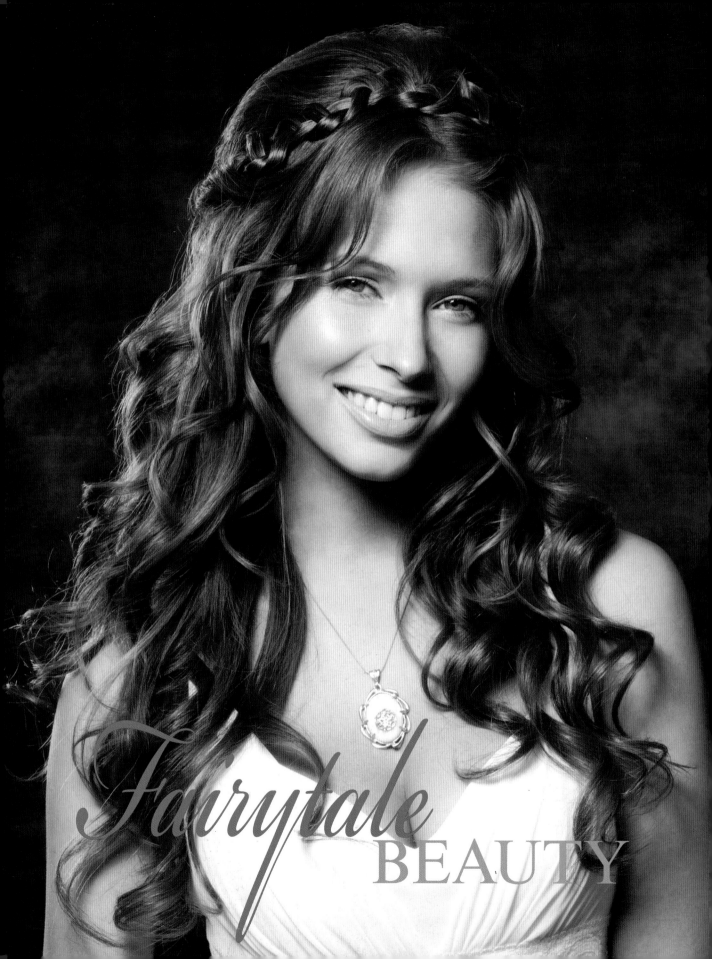

Fairytale
BEAUTY

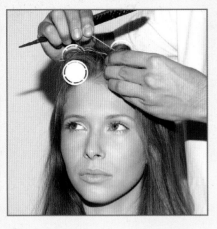

1

1. Wash and blow dry the hair. Make a part down the middle and gather a section of hair at the front of the head, on one side of the part. Roll the hair downwards around a roller and secure. Repeat on the other side of the part.

2. Making your way towards the back of the head, curl another section of hair. This time, use a medium-sized curling iron to roll the hair. Hold the curl in place with a large hair clip.

3. Repeat step 2 by rolling sections of hair all over the head. Spray each rolled section with a little holding spray to hold the curl in place.

4. Allow the curled hair to set for about 10 minutes, then remove the clip from each curl and gently open the curl with your fingers.

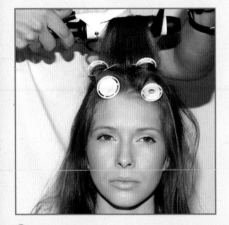

2

Bring fairytale beauty to your special night with this elegant design. Perfectly decorated with a floral hair accessory.

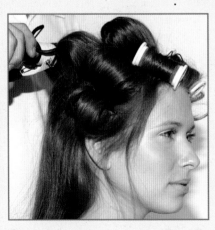

3

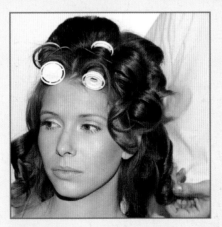

4

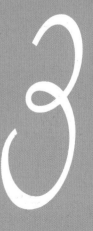

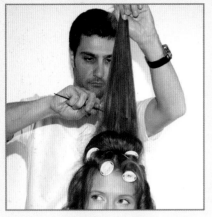

5

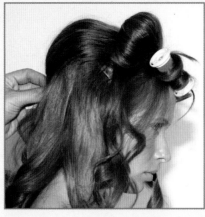

6

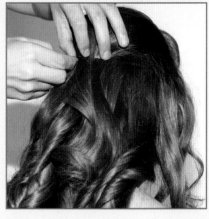

7

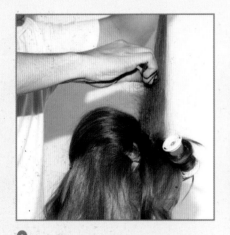

8

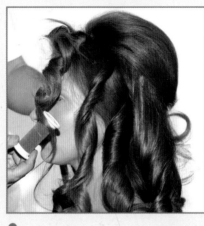

9

5. Gently backcomb each curl to increase volume.

6. Brush out the hair gently without reducing the volume.

7. Mist the hair with holding spray, then draw a curl from the front of the head towards the back and hold it in place with a bobby pin.

8. Take another section of hair from the front, backcomb it at the roots, then draw it towards the back of the head and pin it in place.

9. Gently release the hair at the front of the face from the roller.

10. Gather a section of hair from the front of the head and draw it towards the back. Make sure the curl remains. Pin the hair at the back of the head.

11. Divide a hair extension into three even sections and make a simple braid. Grasp the braid at one end and push the braided hair towards the other end, leaving one part of the hair straight and flat.

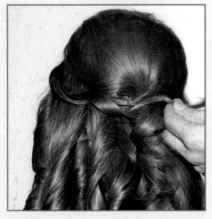

10

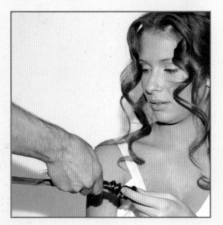

11

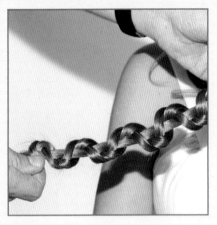

12

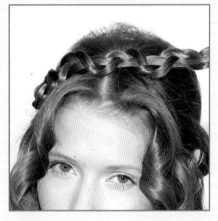

13

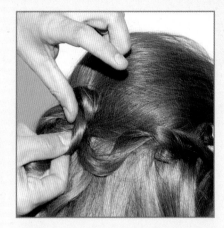

14

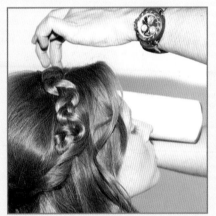

15

12. This technique produces a braid with an interesting texture.

13. Pin one end of the braid above one ear, and bring the braid around the front of the head, like a hair band.

14. Bring the braid towards the back of the head and affix it with bobby pins to the hair at the back of the head.

15. Mist with holding spray to secure the hairstyle. Affix a hair accessory at the back of the head with bobby pins.

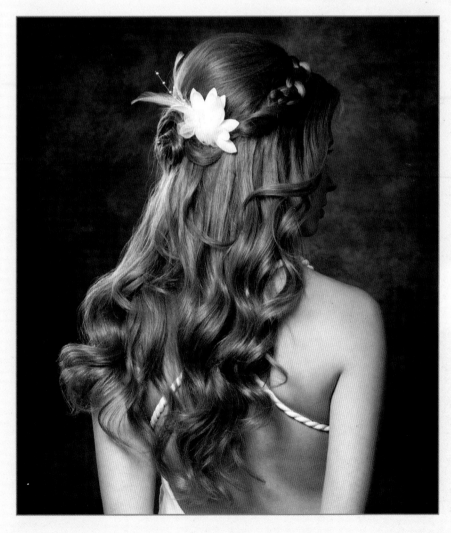

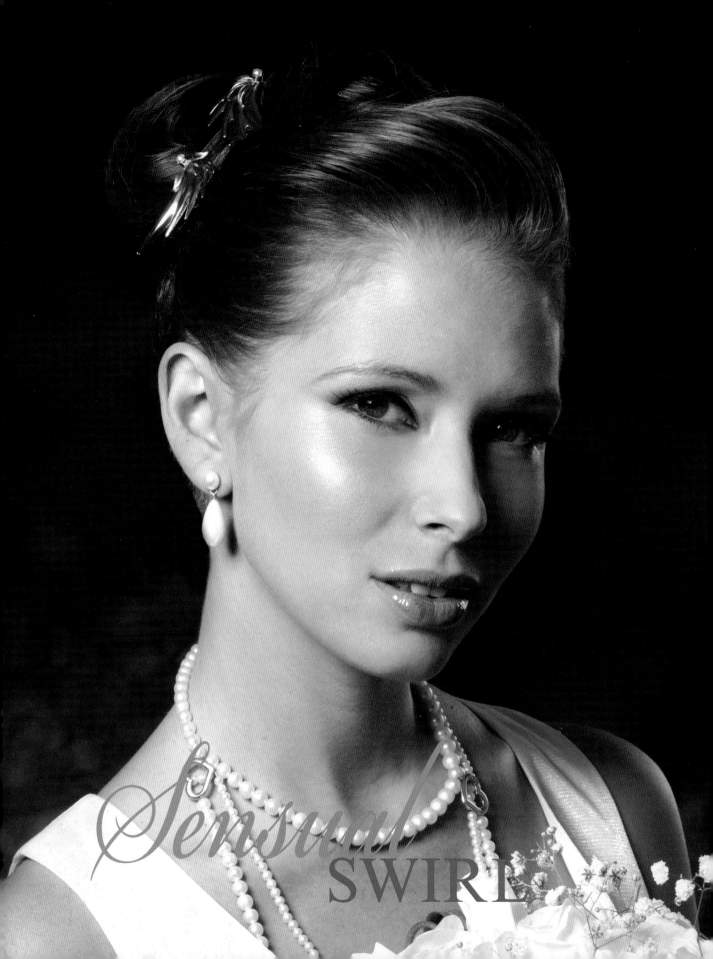
Sensual SWIRL

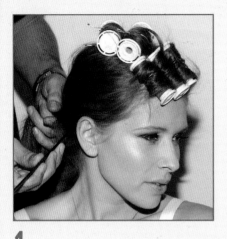

1. Wash and blow dry the hair. Make a relatively large, triangular part above the brow and curl this section of hair with hot rollers.

2. Gather the hair below the curls and above the ear line in a tight ponytail at the back of the head.

3. Brush the loose hair at the back of the head to one side. Secure it with a line of bobby pins that extends upwards from the nape of the neck. For a secure hold, insert the bobby pins in pairs in an X-shape.

4. Brush the rest of the loose hair back over the line of bobby pins. Mist with holding spray to secure it.

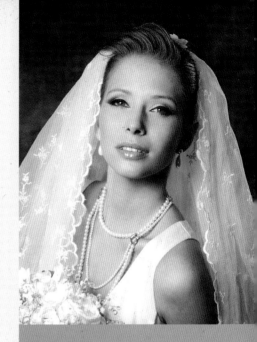

1

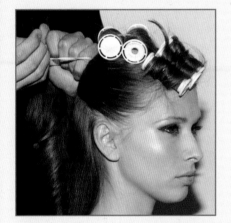

2

This smooth design is wavy, sexy, and elegant. It leaves the neck enticingly visible, so make sure you accessorize with a pretty necklace.

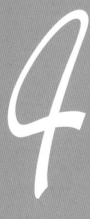

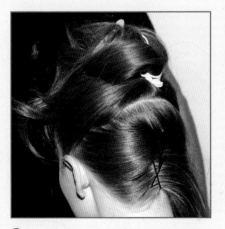

3

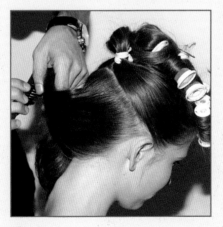

4

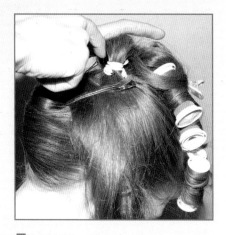

5

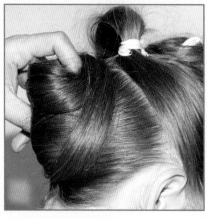

6

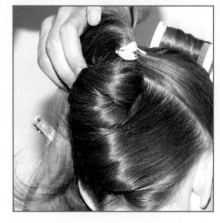

7

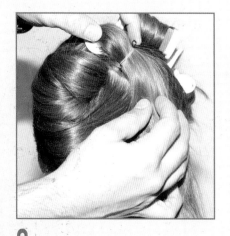

8

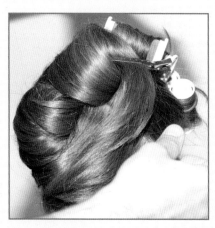

9

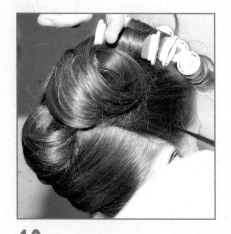

10

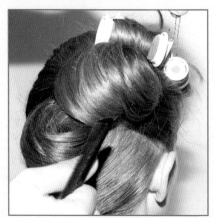

11

5. Roll the hair upwards in a banana twist to cover the line of pins you inserted in step 3. Insert bobby pins close to the scalp to secure the rolled hair firmly.

6. Draw the loose ends of hair over the top of the loop and tuck them inside the loop.

7. Secure this loop of hair with bobby pins.

8. Bring the ponytail you made in step 2 to one side and secure it with bobby pins. Insert the pins in opposite directions (one should be inserted from the top downwards and the other from the bottom upwards). This ensures a secure fit.

9. Fold the hair back in the other direction, wrapping it around to form a loop, and then secure with a large hair clip.

10. Roll the ends of the hair into the center of the loop.

11. Use bobby pins to secure the hairstyle you've created. You may need to use quite a few bobby pins, so insert them gently and carefully to make sure they don't affect the overall look of the hairstyle.

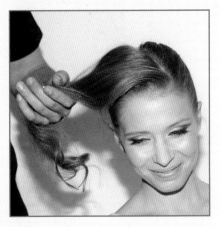 **12**

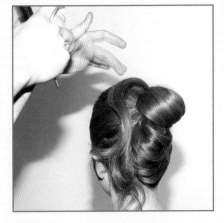 **13**

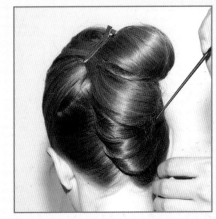 **14**

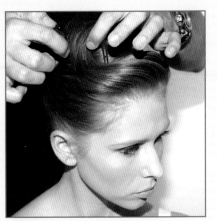 **15**

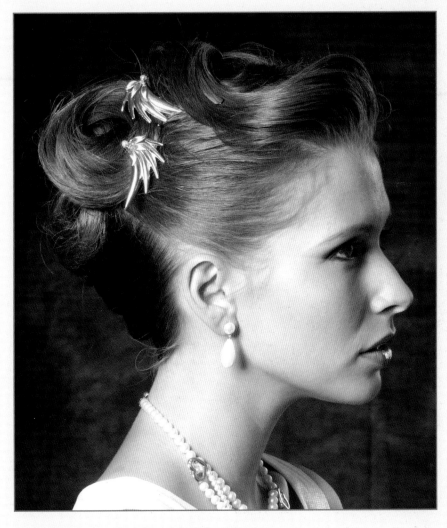

12. Remove the rollers at the front of the hair, lightly brush out the hair and mist with holding spray.

13. Bring the hair backwards, over the hair that has been rolled and pinned at the back of the head. Allow the hair to form a gentle wave and then mist with holding spray.

14. Tuck the section of hair into the rolled hair at the back, so that it blends in smoothly with that hair.

15. Once the holding spray dries, remove the hair clips that were holding the hair temporarily in place. Replace them with bobby pins, inserted close to the scalp.

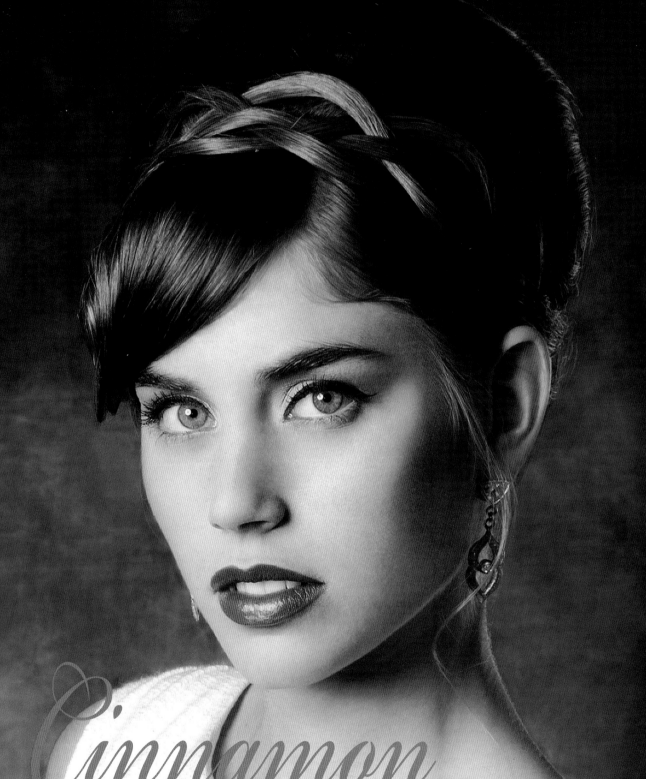

Cinnamon TWIST

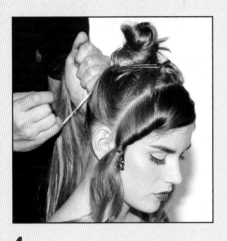

1. Wash and blow dry the hair. Divide the hair into three sections: a front section that extends from ear to ear and up to the brow; a middle section at the crown of the head; and a back section that includes the hair at the back. Gather the hair at the back of the head in a low ponytail.

2. Grasp a 2-inch section of hair immediately above the ponytail and backcomb it at the roots to increase volume.

3. Grasp a similar section immediately above this (closer to the crown) and backcomb it at the roots as well.

4. Draw the backcombed hair backwards and gently brush the exterior so that it is smooth and clean, but without reducing the volume. Mist with holding spray.

1

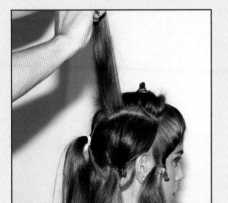

2

This sleek hairstyle is perfect for brides with fine hair. Backcombing adds volume while the twisted bun makes a perfect finish.

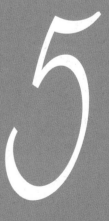

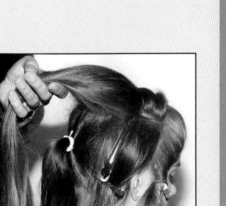

3

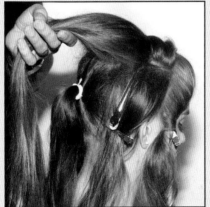

4

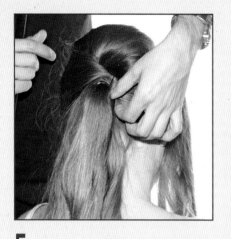

5

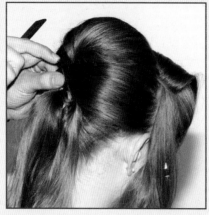

6

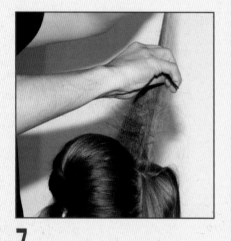

7

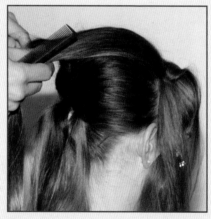

8

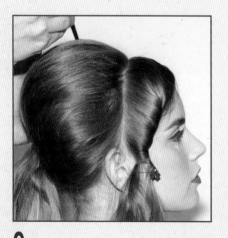

9

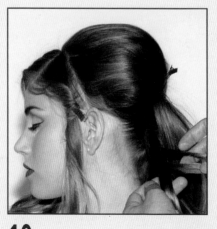

10

5. Twist and pin the backcombed hair just above the ponytail.

6. Repeat this technique to backcomb, brush, and draw back another section of hair at the top of the head. Pin this hair at the top of the ponytail.

7. Repeat this process until you reach the front of the hairline. Make sure you leave the bangs loose. You'll have created volume at the top of the head, while leaving the ends of the hair straight and loose.

8. Gently brush back each section of hair to create a smooth surface. When backcombing the last section of hair, use an especially gentle touch in order to preserve a clean, sleek exterior.

9. Make final adjustments with the end of a tail comb and then mist with holding spray.

10. Draw a section of hair from one side of the ponytail and divide it into four sections. These sections will be used to create a 4-strand braid.

11. To make the braid, bring the rightmost section of hair towards the left by bringing it over the 2nd section, then under the 3rd section. Repeat the same process while moving in the opposite direction. Continue braiding in this way all the way to the end of the hair.

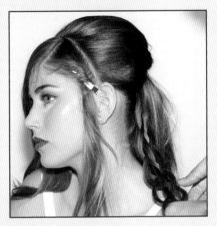

11

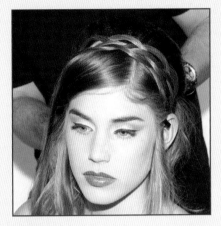

12

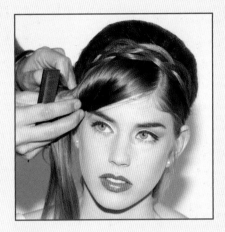

13

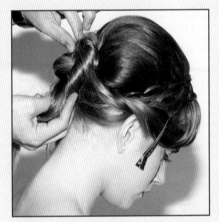

14

12. Bring the braided section of hair up and over the head, like a hair band. Tuck the hair under at the other side and secure with bobby pins.

13. Make a side part with the hair at the brow, then draw the hair to one side of the face and all the way to the back of the head.

14. Twist this section of hair tightly around itself and then wrap it around the base of the ponytail. Secure with bobby pins.

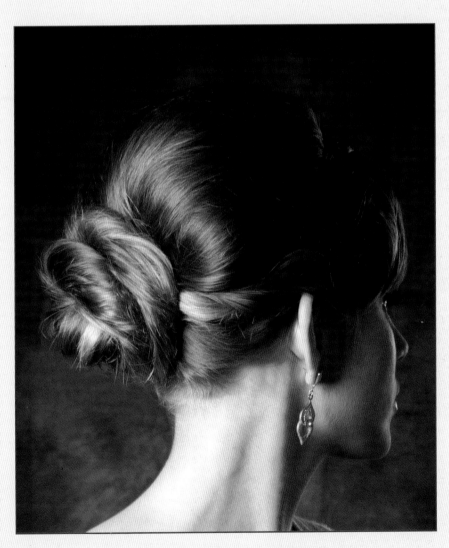

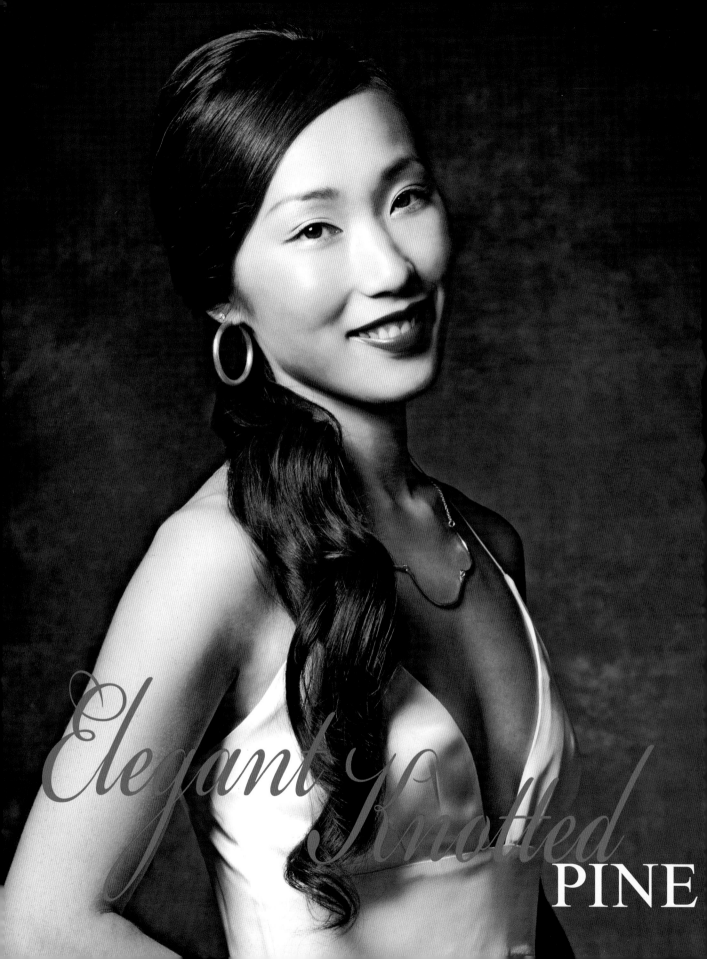

Elegant Knotted
PINE

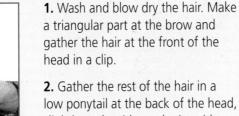

1. Wash and blow dry the hair. Make a triangular part at the brow and gather the hair at the front of the head in a clip.

2. Gather the rest of the hair in a low ponytail at the back of the head, slightly to the side, and mist with holding spray.

3. Secure the hair at the back of the head by making a line of bobby pins, extending from the neck upwards. Make sure the hair is firmly secured by the pins.

4. Place a tail comb on top of the line of bobby pins and brush the hair over the comb.

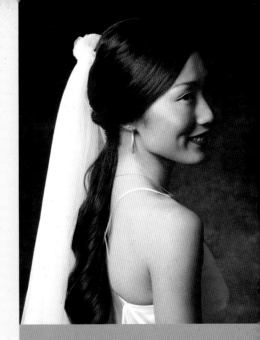

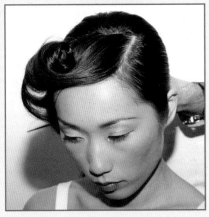

1

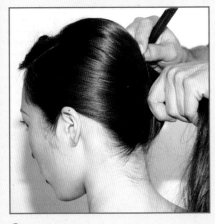

2

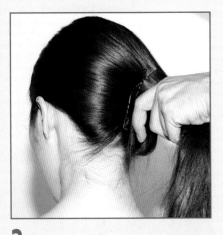

3

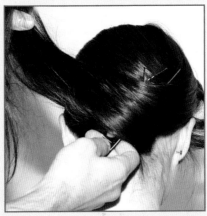

4

This exquisite design creates a gentle wave in naturally straight hair. The knot contrasts beautifully with the ponytail and a tiny flower softens the entire look.

6

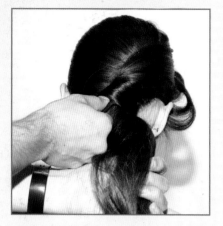

5

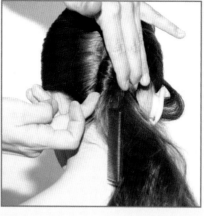

6

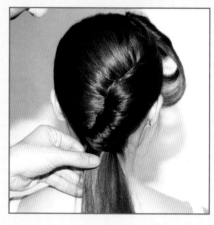

7

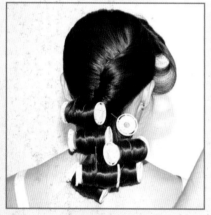

8

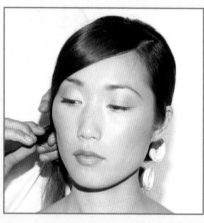

9

5. Wrap the hair over the comb to create a banana shape and arrange the ends of the hair downwards.

6. Insert a large hair clip into the wrapped hair, from the bottom upwards, to secure the twist firmly on the head.

7. Remove the comb from the twist and insert bobby pins all along the seam to reinforce the twist.

8. Roll the ends of hair that extend from the twist around hot rollers. Let the hair set for about 10 minutes.

9. Release the hair at the front of the head from the clip and gently brush it to one side and towards the back.

10. Pin this hair at the top of the twisted hair and mist with holding spray to secure it.

11. Style the ends of the hair upwards.

12. Insert bobby pins some distance from the ends to secure the hair. Draw the ends of the hair downwards over the pins to form a loop. Pin the ends to secure the loop.

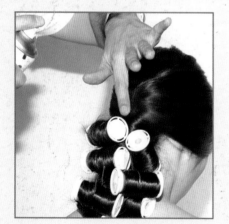

10

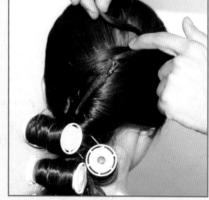

11

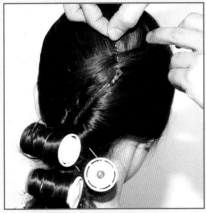

12

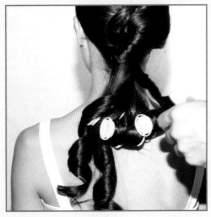

13

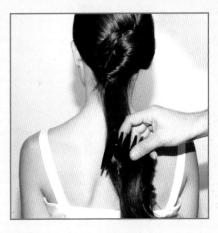

14

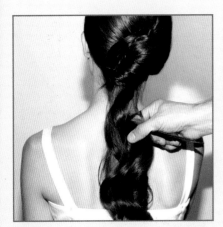

15

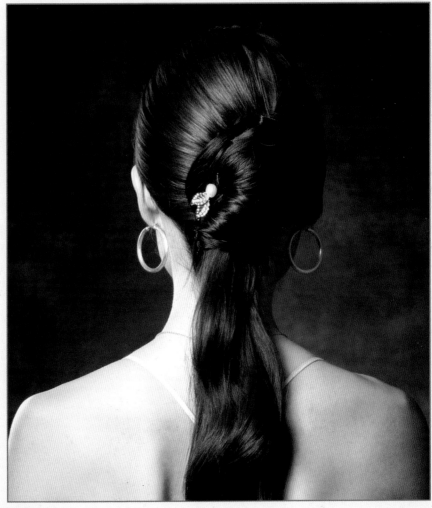

16

13. Release the hair from the rollers, one at a time.

14. Gently brush out the curls with a wide-tooth comb, keeping the waves big and soft.

15. Mist the entire length of the hair with holding spray to preserve the waves for the entire evening.

16. To place the veil, insert the comb directly above the twisted area of the hair design. When removing the veil, make sure you pull out the comb in the exact opposite direction.

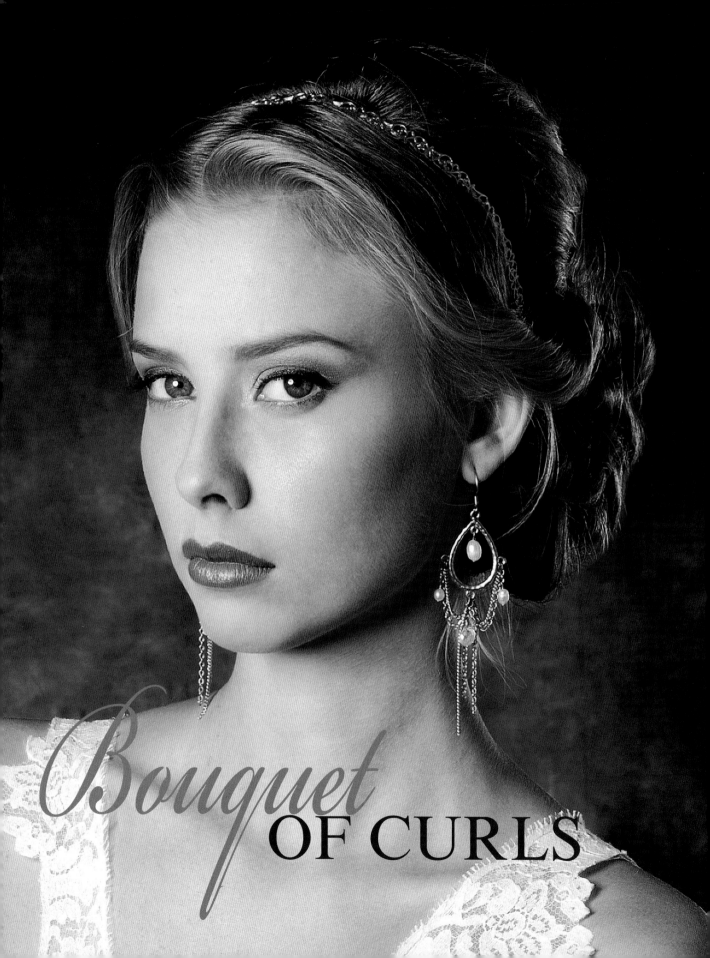

Bouquet
OF CURLS

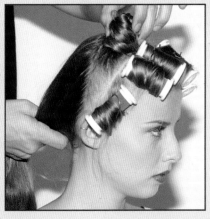

1. Wash and blow dry the hair. Divide the hair into three sections: a front section that includes the hair all around the face; a middle section that extends from ear to ear, over the top of the head; and a back section that includes the hair at the back of the head. Roll the hair around the face in rollers.

2. Gather the hair at the back of the head in a low ponytail and then divide the hair in the ponytail into three even sections.

3. Rub wax onto each of these sections and then braid each section into a simple braid.

4. Backcomb the hair at the crown of the head to increase volume.

Transform your hair into a beautiful bouquet with this feminine design. Add a pretty gold hair band to complete the look.

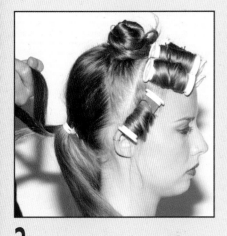

1

2

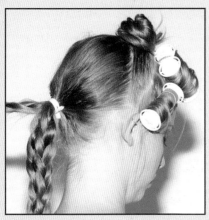

3

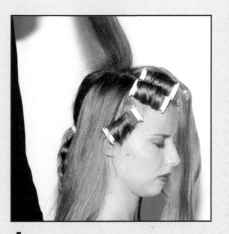

4

7

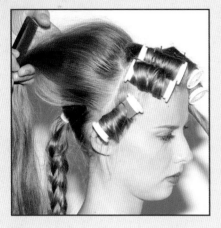

5

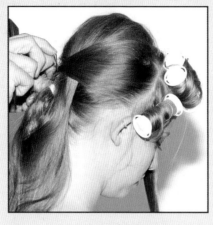

6

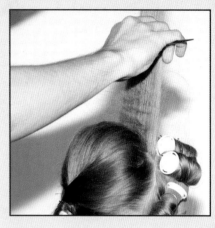

7

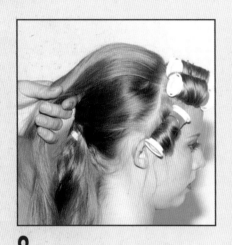

8

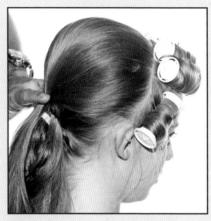

9

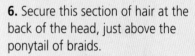

5. Draw the backcombed hair backwards and gently brush the exterior so that it is smooth and clean, but without reducing the volume.

6. Secure this section of hair at the back of the head, just above the ponytail of braids.

7. Gently backcomb the remaining hair at the crown of the head.

8. Draw the hair gently backwards, brush the top to make it smooth and mist with holding spray.

9. Secure the hair at the back, just above the ponytail, with bobby pins.

10. Gently release the rollers from the hair around the face.

11. Very gently brush out the rolled hair to create waves and then mist with holding spray.

12. Gently draw the hair backwards and pin at the back of the head, just above the ponytail. Make sure you don't damage the waves in the hair when you draw it backwards.

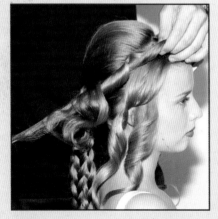

10

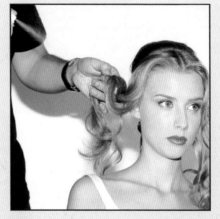

11

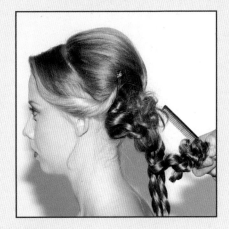

12

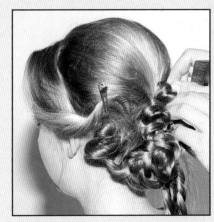

13

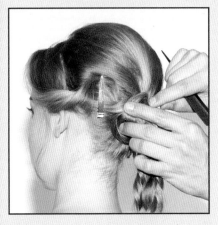

14

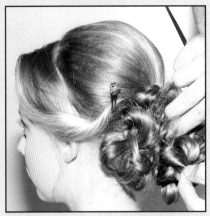

15

13. Grasp the end of one of the braids and push the hair in the braid upwards towards the scalp. This technique loosens the braid and creates an interesting texture.

14. Wrap the loosened braid around the base of the ponytail and secure it with bobby pins.

15. Repeat this technique to loosen the other two braids and create an interesting texture. Twist the braids and secure to the scalp with bobby pins.

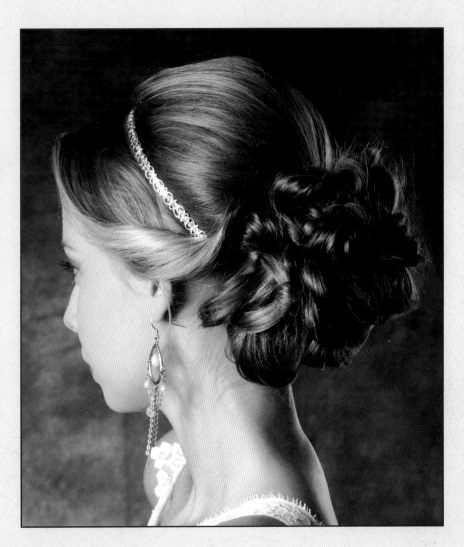

Grecian SPLENDOR

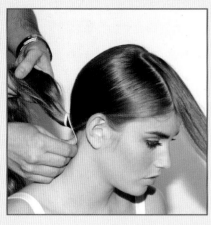

1. Wash and blow dry the hair. Mark off a section, about 1-inch wide, from the crown of the head to the brow and then gather the rest of the hair in a low ponytail at the back of the head.

2. Roll the hair at the front of the head (the hair that isn't in the ponytail) into several curls using a small curling iron. Secure the curls with large hair clips.

3. Twist the hair in the ponytail around itself to form a rope.

4. Roll the twisted hair around itself to form a shape resembling a cinnamon bun. Secure the bun to the head with bobby pins.

1

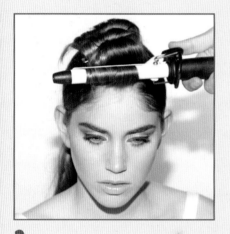

2

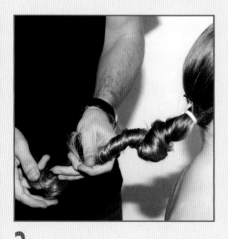

3

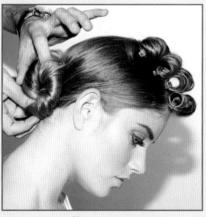

4

Playful waves give this hairstyle its elegant and distinct appearance. Perfect for a bride who loves retro, it's ideal for showing off an interesting hair accessory.

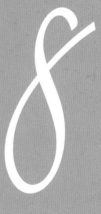

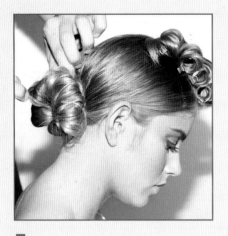

5

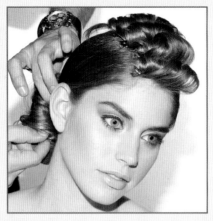

6

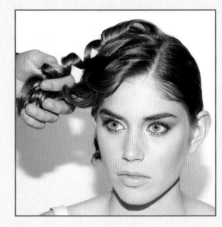

7

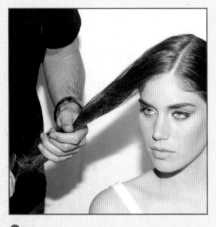

8

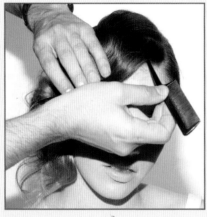

9

5. Draw a few strands of hair out of the twisted roll to create a casual, loose look.

6. Drawing out these strands of hair helps to increase the volume of the hairstyle and gives it a new and interesting texture.

7. Release the hair clips from the curled hair at the front of the head and loosen the curls with your fingers.

8. Gently brush out the hair and bring it to one side of the head.

9. Once the curls are released, the hair will have a gentle wave.

10. Using a metallic butterfly clip, secure the hair at the front of the head just above the wavy part of the hair.

11. Gently brush the hair and style it with your fingers to create another wave.

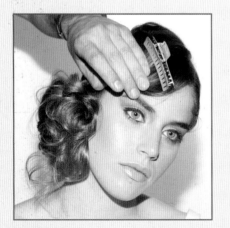

10

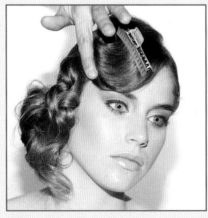

11

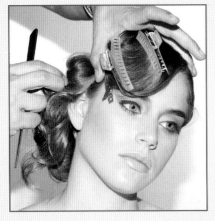

12

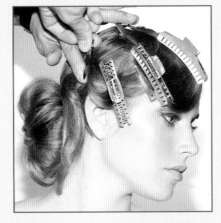

13

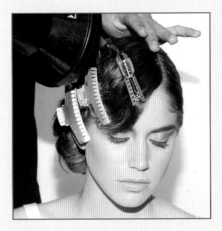

14

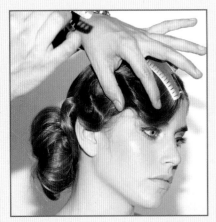

15

12. Insert another clip at the end of the second wave to secure the wave in place.

13. Continue shaping waves in this manner all the way along the length of the hair.

14. Mist the hair with holding spray from a distance of about 8 inches and then dry with a diffuser.

15. Wait for about 10 minutes and then gently remove the clips from the hair. Secure the hairstyle with bobby pins.

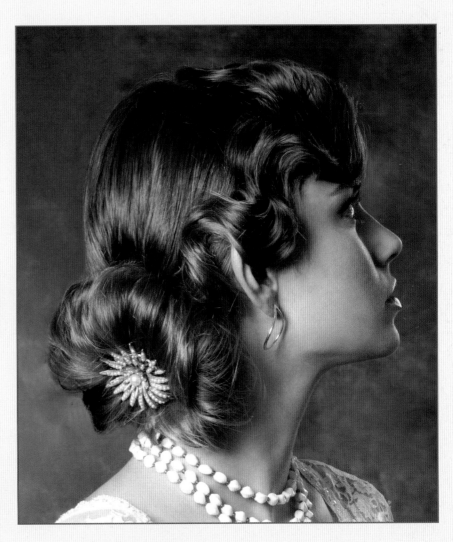

Ravishing WAVES

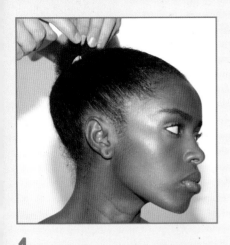

1

1. Wash and blow dry the hair. Brush the hair back and gather it in a high ponytail. Make sure the ponytail is tight.

2. Select hair extensions that match your hair color and affix them to the ponytail.

3. Using a double-barrel curling iron, roll a section of hair between the two prongs to make an X shape.

4. Hold the hair in the curling iron for about 10 seconds and then release gently.

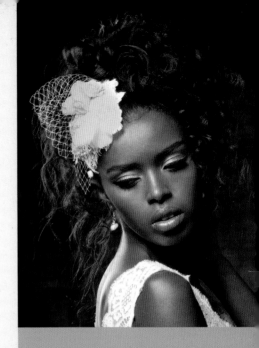

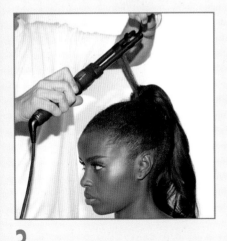

2

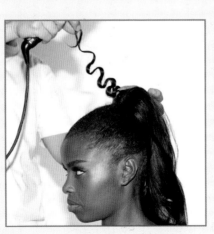

Who says you need long hair to create a long luscious design at your wedding? In this hairstyle, short hair is enhanced with long curled extensions.

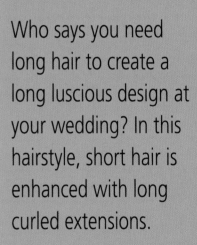

3

4

9

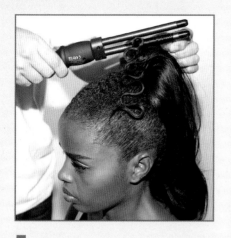

5

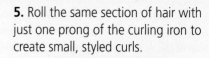
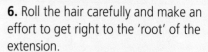
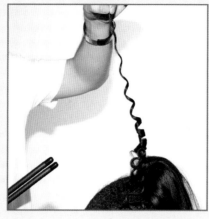

6

5. Roll the same section of hair with just one prong of the curling iron to create small, styled curls.

6. Roll the hair carefully and make an effort to get right to the 'root' of the extension.

7. Continue in this manner, rolling each section of hair first with the double-barrel curling iron and then with a single curling iron, until the entire hair extension has been curled.

8. To ensure that the hairstyle lasts for a long time, mist a little holding spray on each section of hair before curling it.

9. To add volume, grasp a curl at the end and push back the hair towards the roots with your fingers.

10. Push back the hair all the way to the root to give the entire curl a soft natural look.

11. Repeat this technique with all of the curls in the hairstyle, for a really full look.

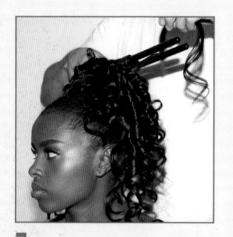

7

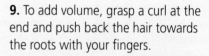
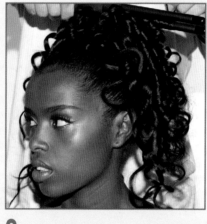

8

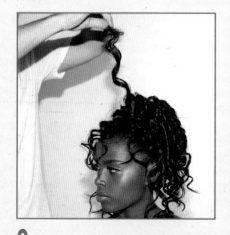

9

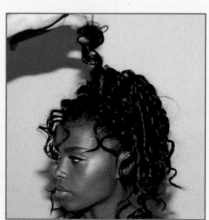

10

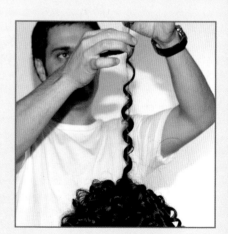

11

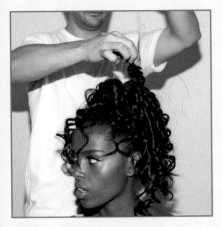

12

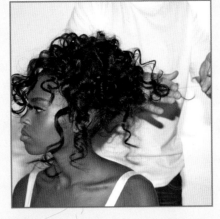

13

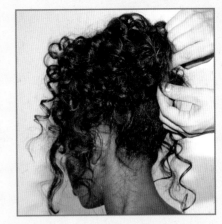

14

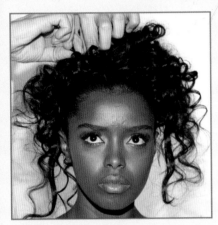

15

12. After pushing back the curls, gently pull it back to its previous state.

13. Repeat this technique with all the hair.

14. To create a playful hairstyle, use bobby pins to secure the hair all around the head

15. Use a mirror when pinning the curls. In this way you can ensure that the curls you pin at the back create the effect you want when they are seen from the front.

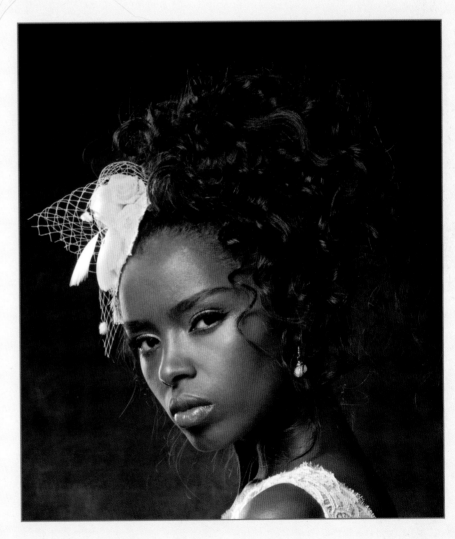

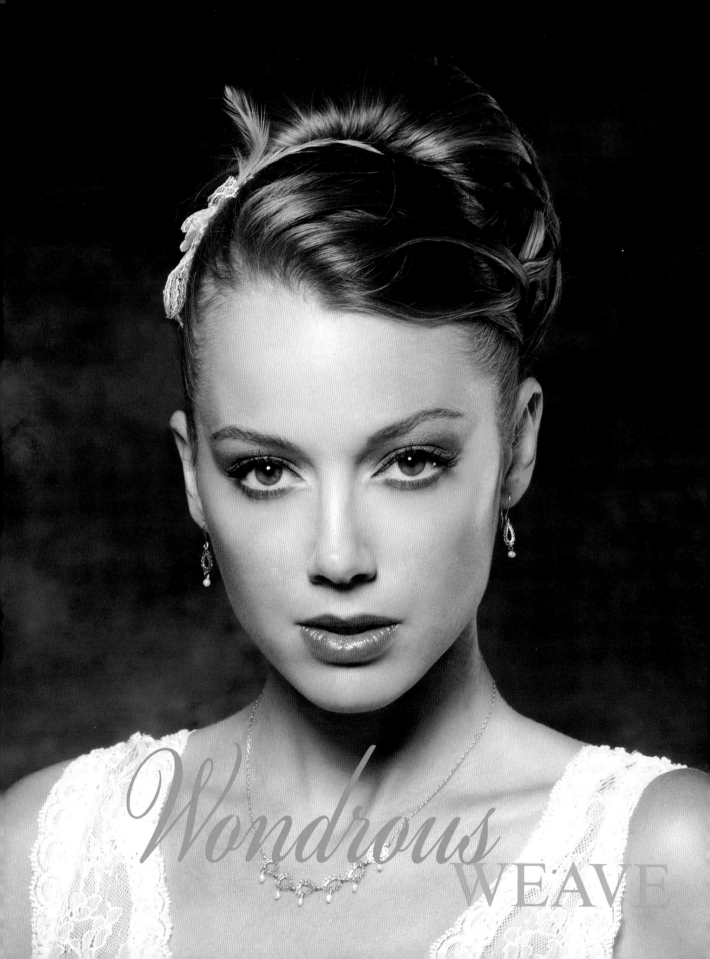

Wondrous WEAVE

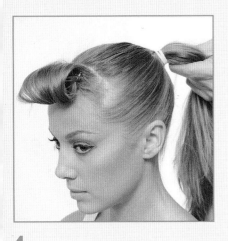

1

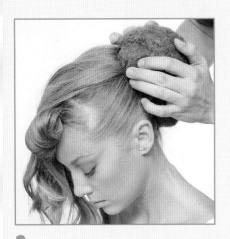

2

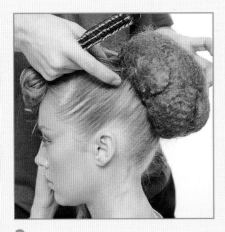

3

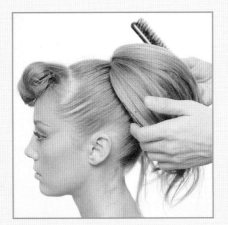

4

1. Wash and blow dry the hair. Make a part that separates the bangs from the rest of the hair. Secure the bangs at the front of the head and collect the rest of the hair in a ponytail at the back.

2. Flip the hair in the ponytail over the top of the head, and affix a hair wrap immediately below the base of the ponytail using bobby pins.

3. Pin the end of the ponytail to the scalp, close to the bottom of the hair wrap, by inserting bobby pins in an X shape.

4. Gently draw the hair in the ponytail over the hair wrap. Gently brush out half the hair, so that it covers half the hair wrap.

5. Hold the brushed hair over the hair wrap at the bottom. Use a tail comb to draw up several small sections of hair from the ponytail. Brush the hair below these lifted sections and mist with holding spray.

Increasing the volume of your hair is easy with a strategically placed hair wrap. In this design, it's accented with a few delicately woven strands of hair.

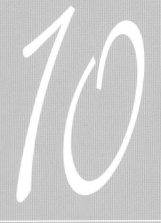

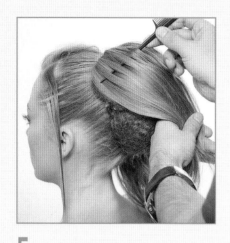

5

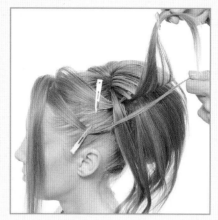

6

6. Draw out a small section of hair from the bangs and bring it to the back of the head. Draw the section over the hair wrap, so that it is under the sections of hair you lifted in step 5, but over the hair wrap. Pin this section of hair on the other side of the hair wrap (or to the scalp, if it reaches that far). Bring down the sections of hair that were lifted in step 5, and then draw up contrasting sections of hair from the ponytail. Draw another section of hair from the bangs.

7. Repeat the technique you used in step 6 to place the strand of hair from the bangs over the ponytail. Note that this time, opposite sections of hair will cover the strand from the bangs. Secure the strand at the back of the head with a bobby pin.

8. Gently brush the hair covering the hair wrap and then mist with a little holding spray to secure it.

9. Repeat this process with additional strands of hair that you have drawn from the bangs to create a woven look on the hair wrap. Mist with holding spray.

10. Make sure that you weave each strand of hair neatly, since this helps to show off the pattern.

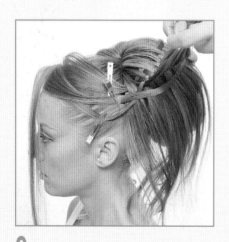

7

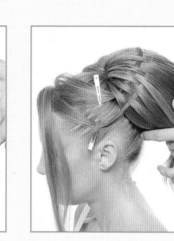

8

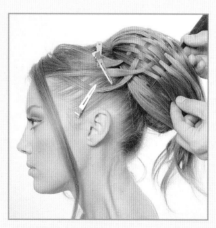

9

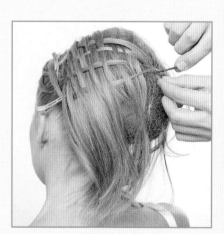

10

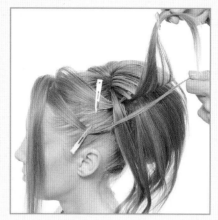

11

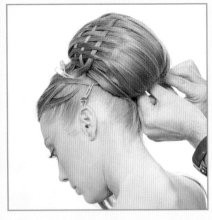

12

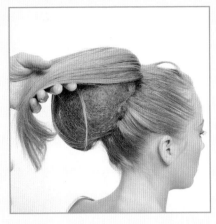

13

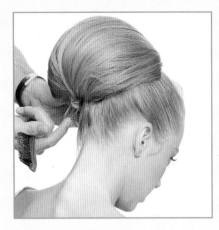

14

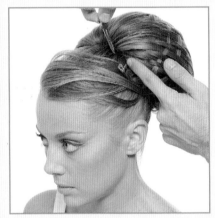

15

11. After all the bangs have been woven into the hair covering the hair wrap, gather all of them together at the back of the head and secure using bobby pins.

12. Gently brush the ends of the hair over the hair wrap, roll the ends, and secure them with a bobby pin, close to the scalp.

13. Brush out the remaining half of the ponytail over the hair wrap. Mist the hair with holding spray to secure it over the hair wrap.

14. Roll the ends of this section of hair and secure with bobby pins, close to the scalp.

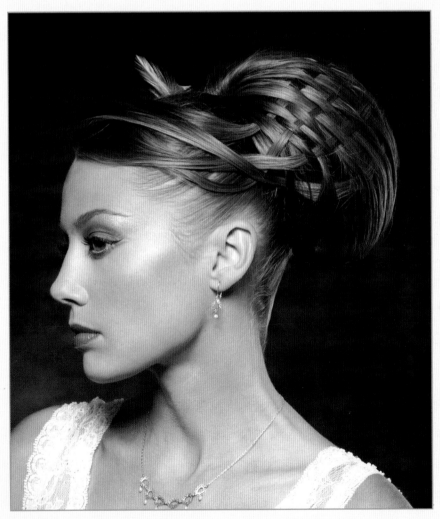

15. When the hairstyle is just right, gently remove the clips and mist with holding spray to secure it.

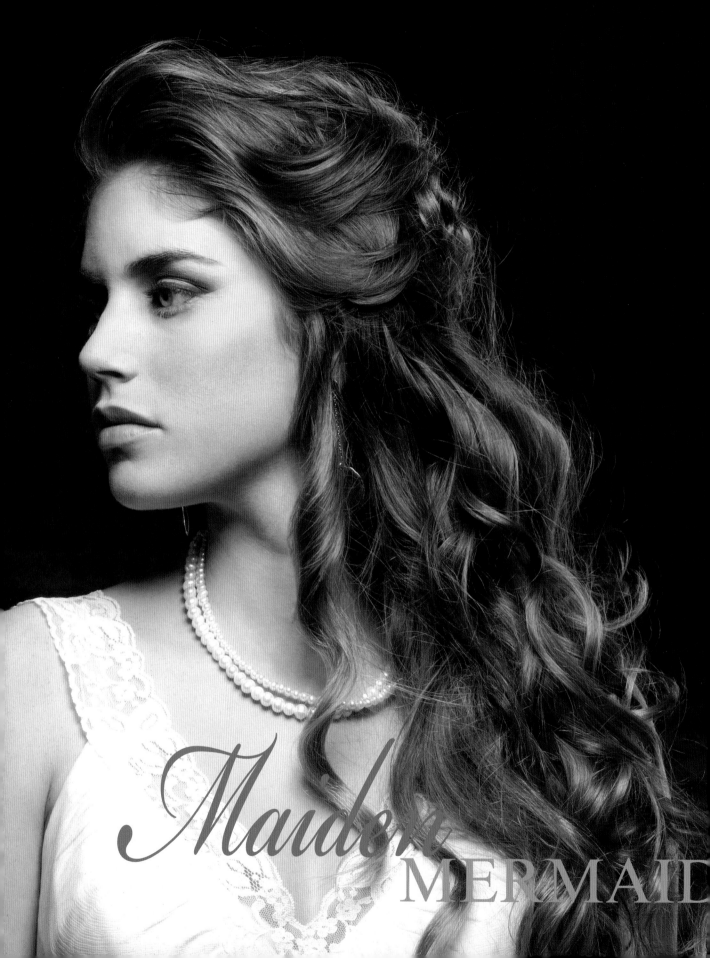

Maiden
MERMAID

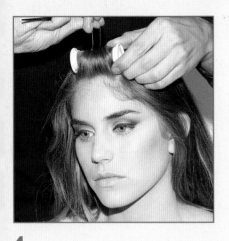

1. Wash and blow dry the hair. Roll the hair at the front of the head with hot rollers.

2. Curl the hair at the back of the head with a large curling iron.

3. Use hair clips to secure each of the sections of hair you curled with the curling iron.

4. Repeat this technique with the rest of the hair.

1

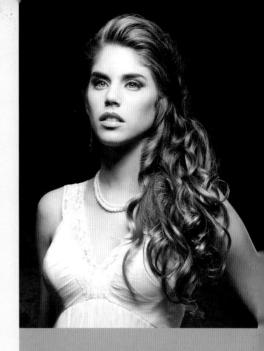

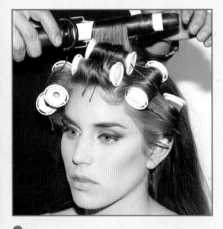

2

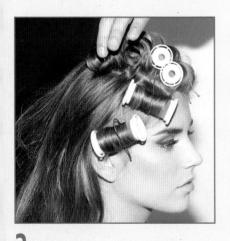

3

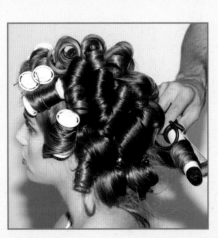

4

In this romantic hairstyle, several sections of hair are whirled together beautifully to create an unusual decoration. Naturally beautiful.

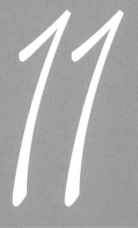

11

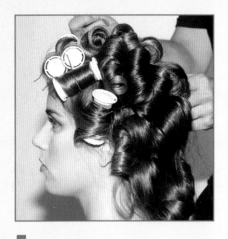

5

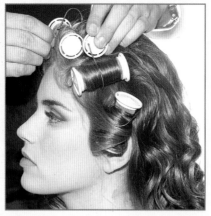

6

5. Let the curls set for about 10 minutes, then release the hairclips and let the curls loosen.

6. Gently release the rollers around the face and use your fingers to gently open the curls into waves.

7. Draw two sections of wavy hair from the front of the head towards the back. Secure the two sections in the middle of the head with bobby pins, inserted in an X shape. This serves as the base of the hairstyle.

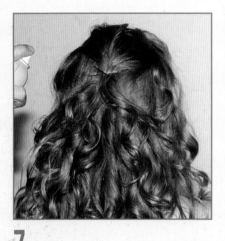

7

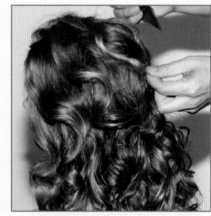

8

8. Using a wide-tooth comb, work on one section of hair at a time. Brush each section and draw it back, from the front of the head to the back. Pin the sections of hair to the base of the hairstyle in a way that preserves the curls.

9. Make sure you retain the waves in the hair as you draw the sections from the front of the head to the back.

10. Gather the hair at the back of the head, to the right of the hairstyle base.

11. To create an asymmetrical look, draw more sections of hair towards the right side of the head. Mist with holding spray to secure.

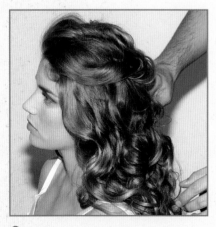

9

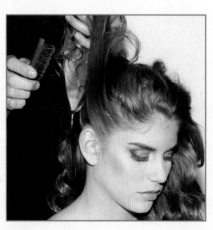

10

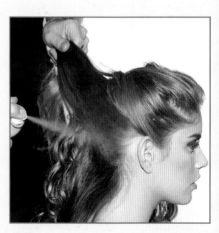

11

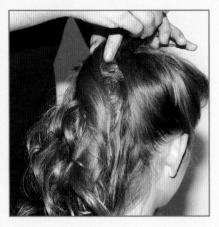

12

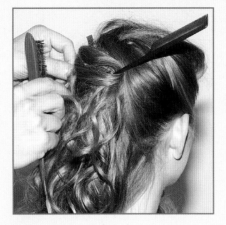

13

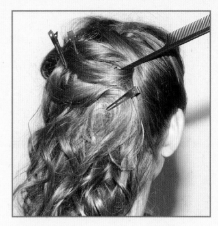

14

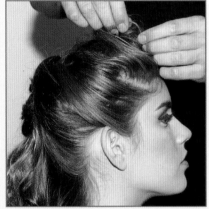

15

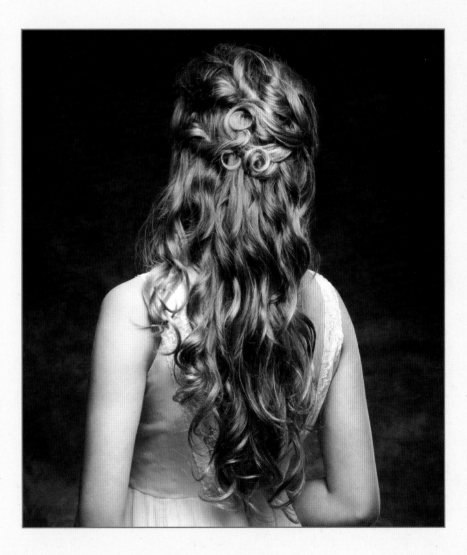

12. Insert a rattail comb into the base of the hairstyle and draw the section of hair around the comb.

13. Secure the hair with hair clips, then insert another comb (or remove the previous comb and reuse it) into another point in the hairstyle, and draw the hair around it (in the other direction).

14. Mist the hair with a little holding spray and wait a few minutes for it to set. Insert bobby pins to secure the hair and then remove the hair clips.

15. To finish the hairstyle, draw out a few sections of hair to create a soft, natural look.

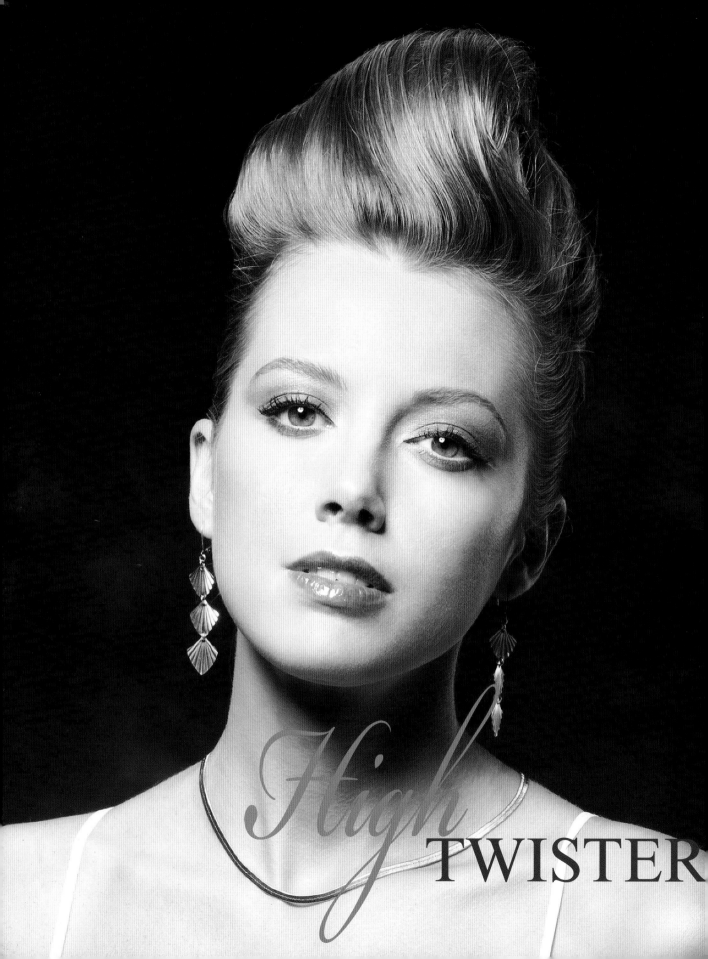

High TWISTER

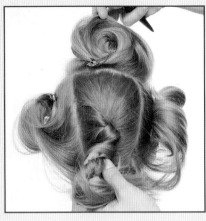

1

1. Wash and blow dry the hair. Make a rectangular part at the back of the head to divide the hair into four groups. Secure the hair in each group with elastic bands.

2. Mark off a section of hair, about 2 inches wide, at the nape of the neck and then backcomb it at the roots to increase volume.

3. Work your way up the back of the head, backcombing similarly sized sections of hair, all the way to the top of the head.

4. Repeat this technique to backcomb the hair on one side of the head. Make sure you backcomb the hair at the roots and about 8 inches along the length of the hair, but do not backcomb the ends.

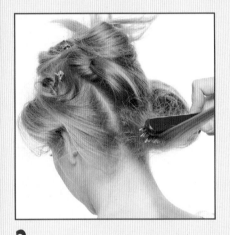

2

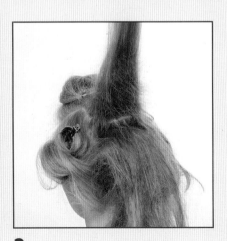

3

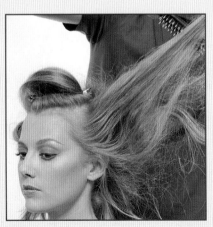

4

This unmistakable hairstyle is just right for the bride who wants to be chic and stylish on her wedding day.

12

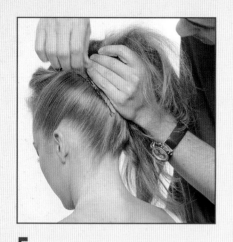

5

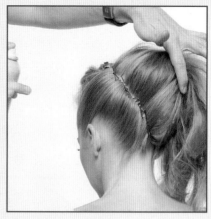

6

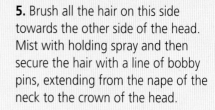

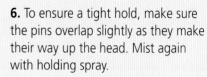

5. Brush all the hair on this side towards the other side of the head. Mist with holding spray and then secure the hair with a line of bobby pins, extending from the nape of the neck to the crown of the head.

6. To ensure a tight hold, make sure the pins overlap slightly as they make their way up the head. Mist again with holding spray.

7. Move to the other side of the head and mist with holding spray. Brush the hair on this side towards the other side of the head.

8. Bring the hair over the line of pins and twist it halfway upwards to form a banana shape. Hold the twisted hair in place with bobby pins.

9. Brush the edges of the twisted hair into the other hair, so that they blend in smoothly.

10. Release the hair at the front of the head and backcomb it at the roots to increase volume.

11. After the hair has been backcombed, brush it out and mist with holding spray for a smooth look.

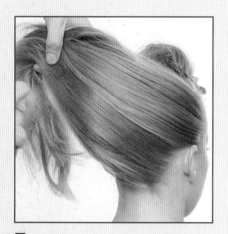

7

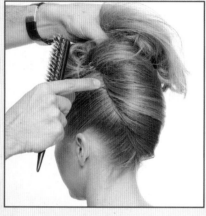

8

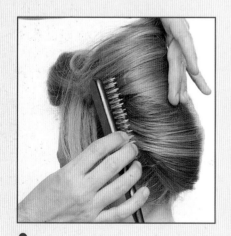

9

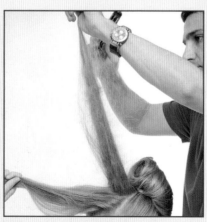

10

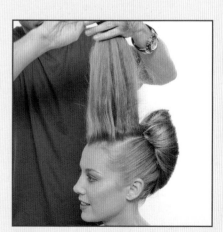

11

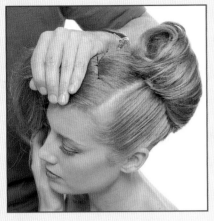

12

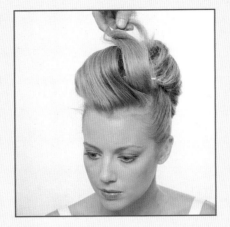

13

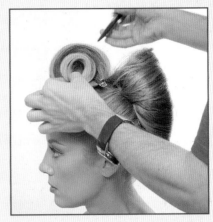

14

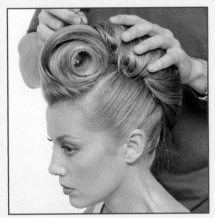

15

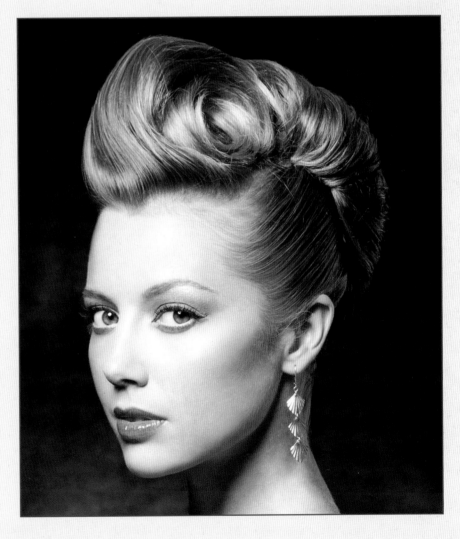

12. Bring the hair forward and insert bobby pins at an angle, from the brow to the ear line, in order to make a base for gathering the hair at the front.

13. Brush the hair upwards to increase the height and then roll the hair over the line of pins to create a thick roll. Secure with a hair clip.

14. Tuck the ends of the hair inside the roll you just made and adjust them so that they fit neatly inside.

15. To complete the hairstyle, draw the twisted hair at the back towards the gathered hair at the front and secure with bobby pins.

Exquisitely WRAPPED

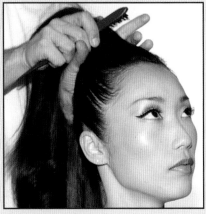

1. Wash and blow dry the hair. Divide the hair into front and back sections by making a part over the crown of the head.

2. Gather the hair at the front of the head in a high ponytail. Gather the hair at the back of the head in a low ponytail.

3. Divide the hair in the back ponytail into three sections. Rub a bit of wax onto each section of the ponytail.

4. Begin braiding the hair in the back ponytail.

1

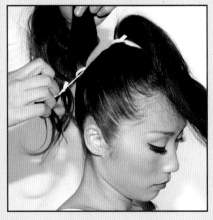

2

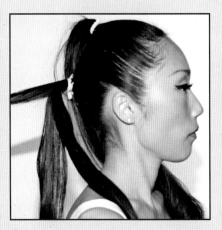

3

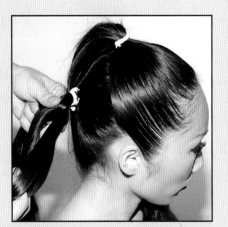

4

Transform naturally straight hair into a textured treasure of wrapped braids. Add a decorative hair band to complete the look.

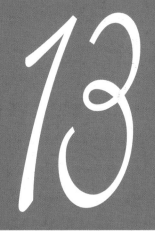

13

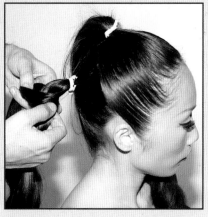

5

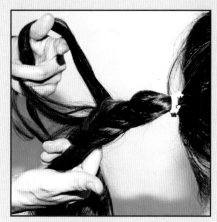

6

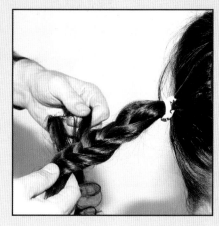

7

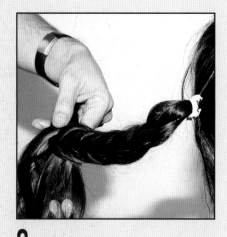

8

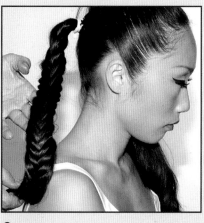

9

5. At every stage of the braid, draw one-third of each section of hair towards the middle of the braid.

6. As you advance with the braid, you'll see a unique design take shape.

7. Continue separating one-third of each section of hair each time you integrate another section into the braid.

8. As you progress with the braid, you'll notice that you have already separated sections of hair from the braid and they won't need to be divided into thirds anymore.

9. The resulting braid has many sections and a really interesting texture. When you reach the end of the braid, secure it with an elastic band.

10. Repeat this braiding technique with the top ponytail and secure it at the end with an elastic band.

11. Grasp the end of the top braid, hold a small section of the hair in your hand, and gently begin pushing the braid up.

12. Continue pushing up the braid until it tightens and is close to the scalp.

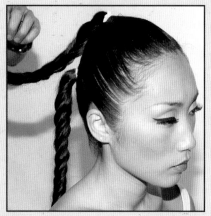

10

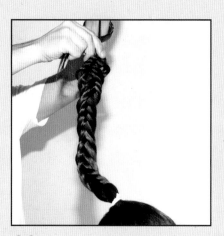

11

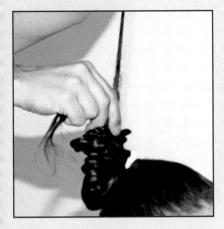

12

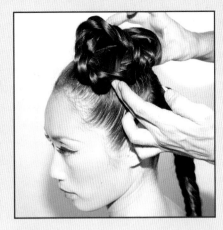

13

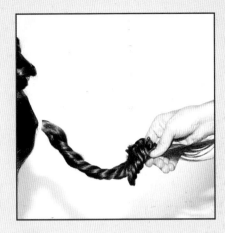

14

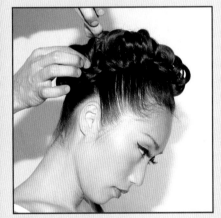

15

13. Twist the braid around the elastic band at the base to conceal the elastic band and create the desired shape. Secure the braid with bobby pins.

14. Hold the end of the second braid in the same way and push the braid up towards the scalp.

15. Twist the second braid around the base of the elastic band, concealing it and forming a harmonious design with the first braid. Secure the braid with bobby pins. To complete the hairstyle, gently draw out some of the sections of hair to increase volume.

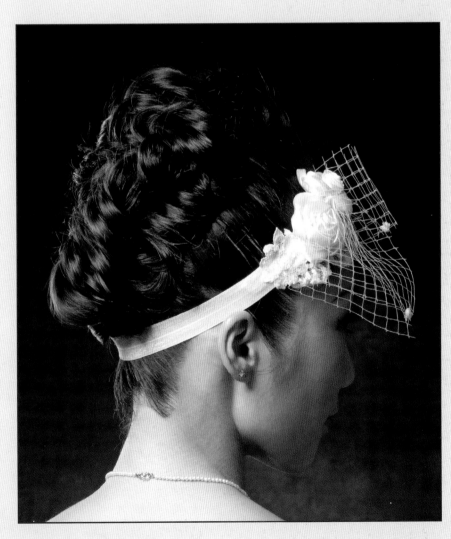

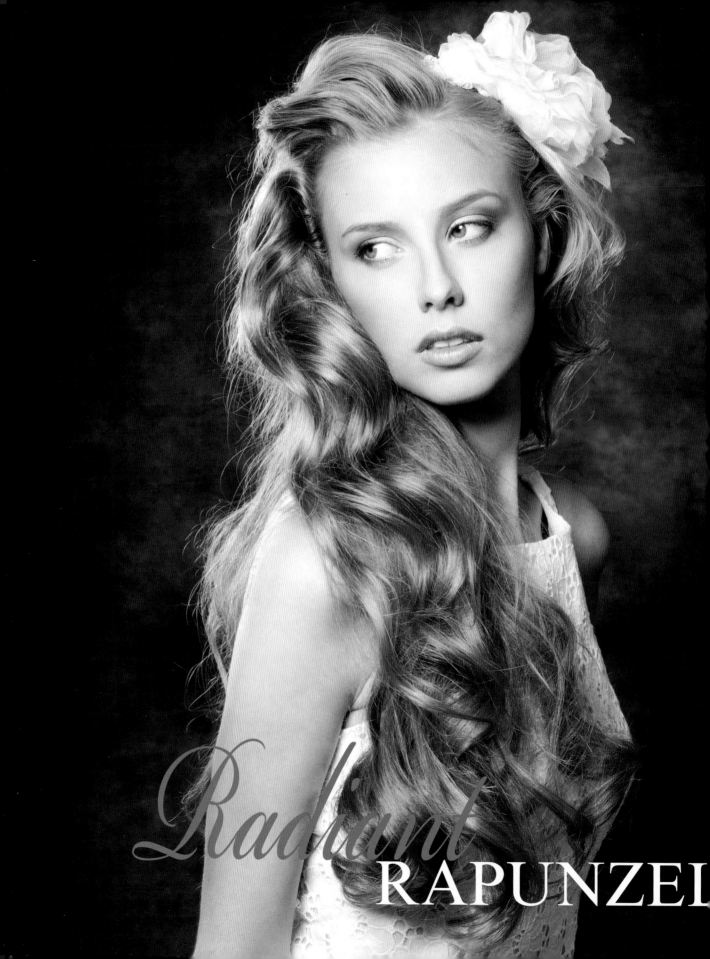

Radiant RAPUNZEL

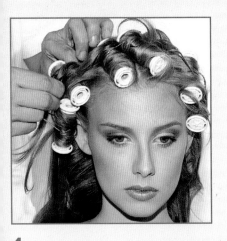

1

1. Wash and blow dry the hair. Roll the hair around the face with hot rollers. Mist the rolled hair with holding spray.

2. Using a curling iron, curl the hair at the back of the head, all the way to the crown.

3. Let the rolled hair set for about 10 minutes and then gently remove the rollers.

4. Gently open the curls with your fingers.

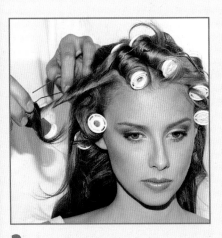

2

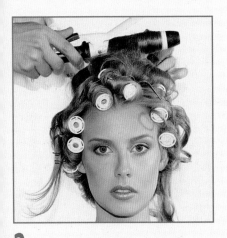

3

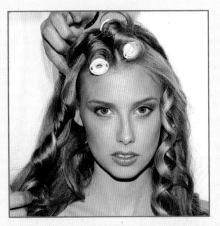

4

Bring even more magic to your evening with this charming hairstyle. Beautiful and indulgent, it's perfect for displaying a striking, bold hair accessory.

14

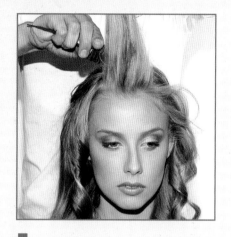

5

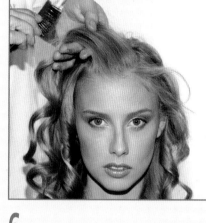

6

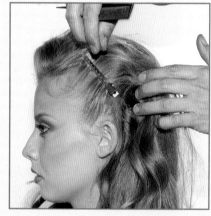

7

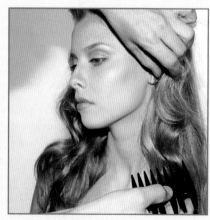

8

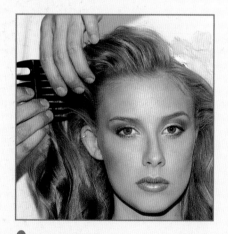

9

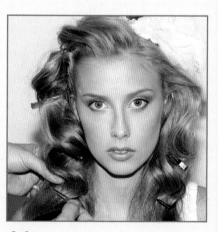

10

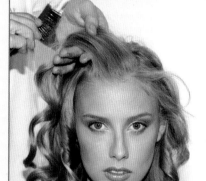

11

5. To increase volume at the top of the face, gently backcomb the hair at the roots.

6. Draw this hair backwards and very gently brush the part of the hair that will be visible when it is drawn backwards. Make sure you brush the hair gently so as not to reduce the volume at the roots.

7. Draw the hair loosely backwards and secure in place with bobby pins. Make sure you retain height at the top of the face.

8. Gently brush back the hair at the sides of the face. Use a small hair comb to secure the hair while creating volume.

9. Gently brush the curled hair into waves using a wide-tooth comb.

10. Open the curls with the comb or your fingers until you achieve the desired effect.

11. Arrange the waves as desired and use hair clips to hold them in place.

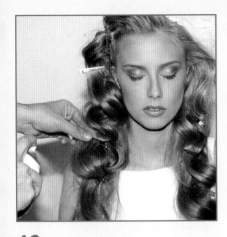

12

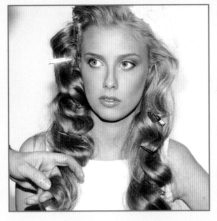

13

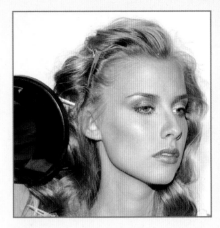

14

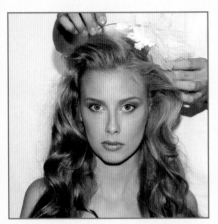

15

12. Mist the hair with holding spray at a distance of about 8 inches.

13. Make sure you work very gently when shaping the hair, so that the waves stay soft and gentle.

14. Heat the hair with a diffuser and then let it cool for about 10 minutes. When the hair has set, carefully remove the hair clips.

15. To finish the look, insert a flower accessory at the back of the head.

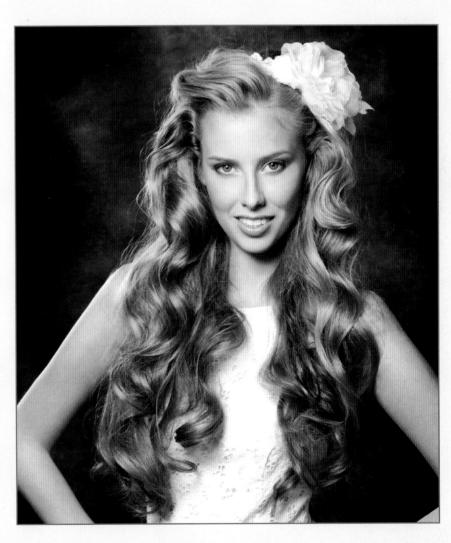

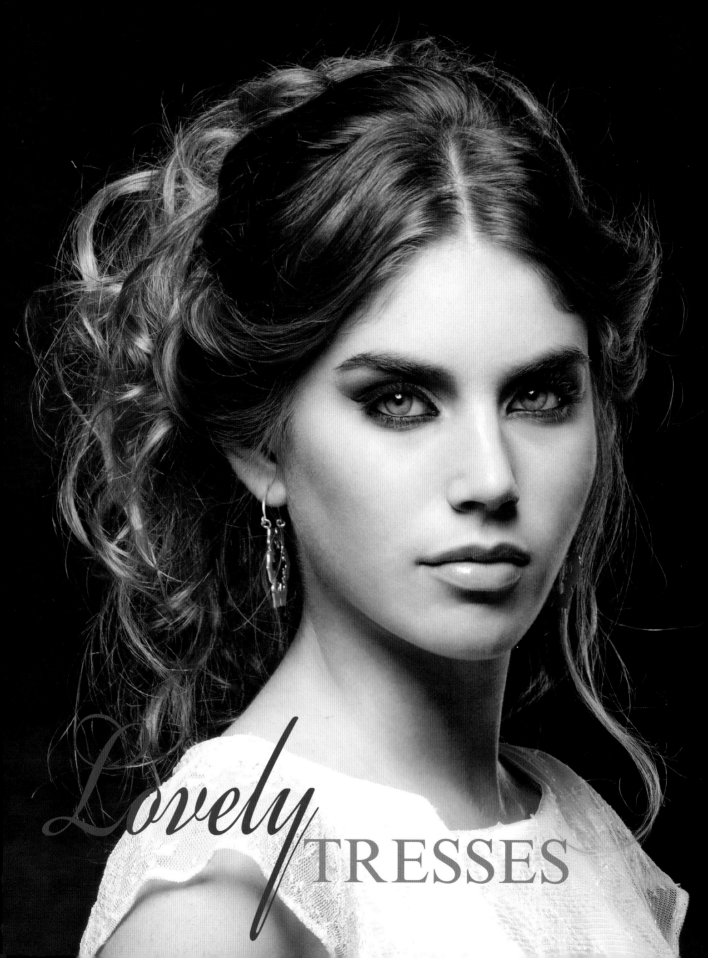

Lovely TRESSES

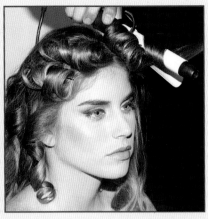

1. Wash and blow dry the hair. Using a medium-sized curling iron, curl the hair around the face. Secure each curl with a hair clip.

2. Continue to curl the rest of the hair, but there is no need to secure the curls with hair clips.

3. Draw a section of hair from above each ear towards the back of the head and secure the two sections together with an elastic band.

4. Release the hair clips from the curls around the face and gently loosen the curls with your fingers.

1

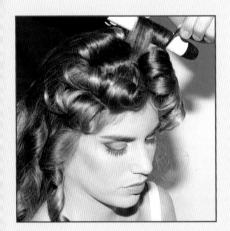

2

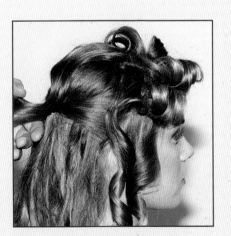

This pretty hairstyle features twisted sides that sweep gracefully upwards at the back. Playful and pretty, it's perfect for either a bride or a bridesmaid.

3

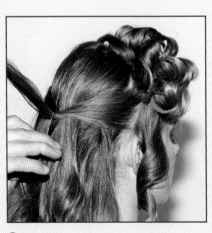

4

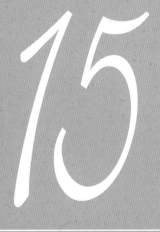

15

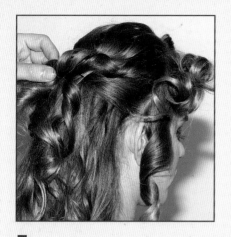

5

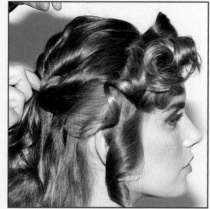

6

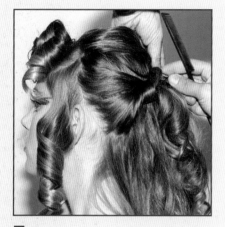

7

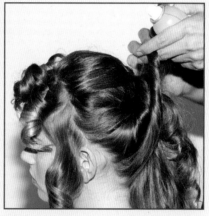

8

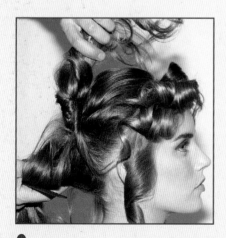

9 —

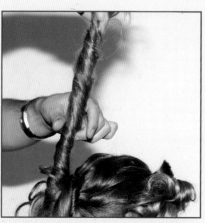

10

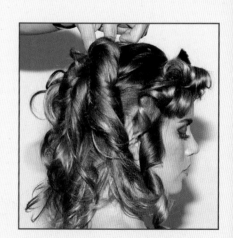

11

5. Draw the curls from the front of the head to the back and secure with bobby pins. Make sure you don't damage the curls as you draw them backwards.

6. Mist each curl with a little holding spray before drawing it backwards and pin all of the curls at the same area at the back of the head. This will serve as the base of the hairstyle.

7. Make sure you don't draw the hair backwards too tightly.

8. Once all the hair from the front has been gathered at the back, begin twisting, lifting, and pinning the hair at the back of the head.

9. Separate the pinned hair from the hair that is still loose.

10. Roll the loose hair at the back of the head upwards and twist it gently in a circular motion.

11. Pin the twisted section of hair at the base (you created it with the sections of hair you drew backwards from the front of the head).

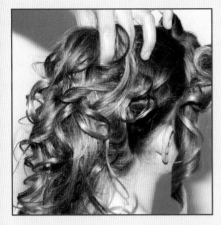

12

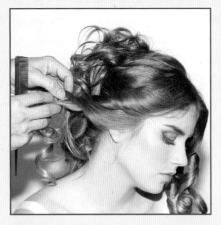

13

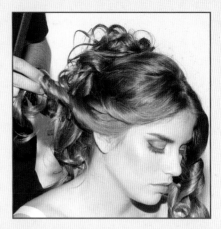

14

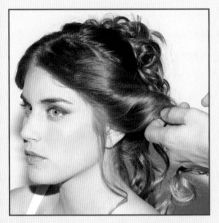

15

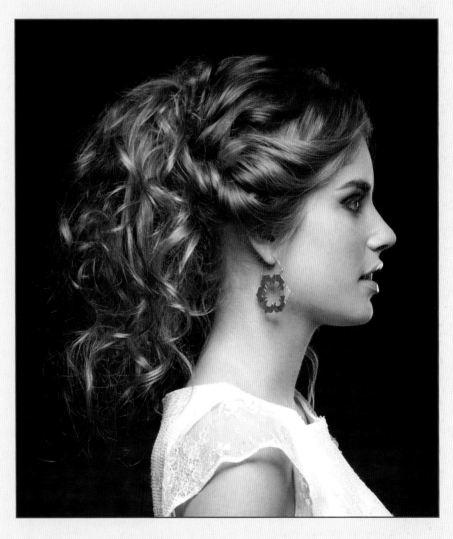

12. Secure the hair at the base of the collected hair in a way that looks loose and natural.

13. Draw two curled sections of hair gently backwards from one side of the front of the head. Twist the sections as you draw them back so that they twist together.

14. It's important to leave the hair soft and wavy around the face, but twisted while securing it at the back.

15. Repeat this technique on the other side of the head. Mist the entire hairstyle with holding spray to secure it.

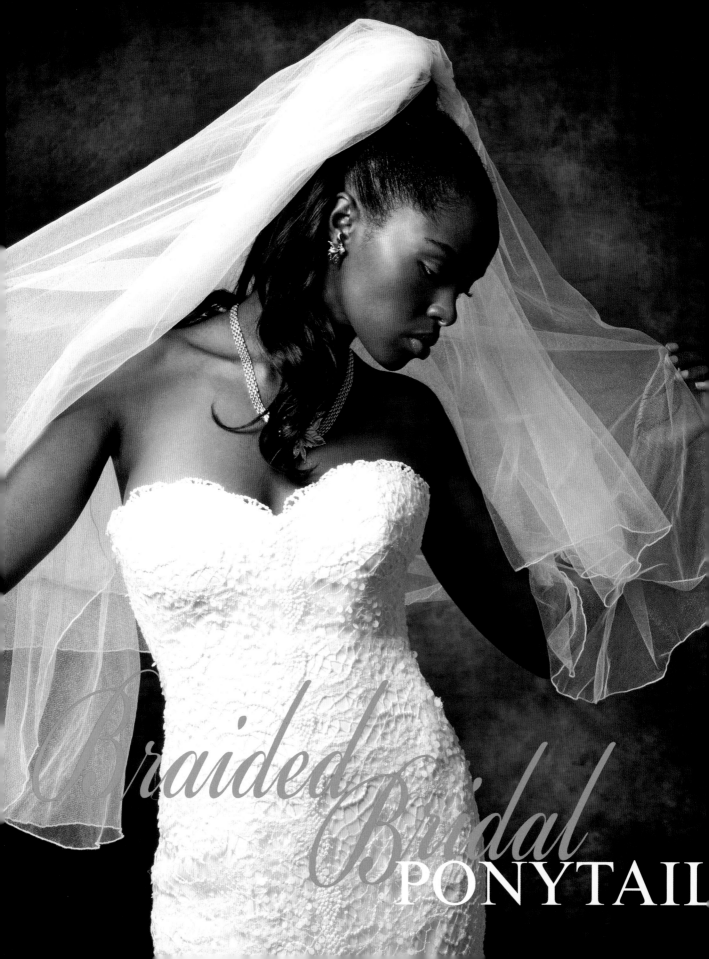

Braided Bridal PONYTAIL

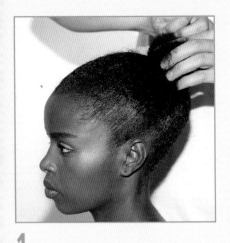

1. Wash and blow dry the hair. Brush the hair back and gather it in a high ponytail.

2. Select a hairnet that matches the color of the hair and wrap it around the ponytail.

3. If the hair is curly, mist the hair with holding spray and blow dry as you brush it backwards to create a really smooth surface.

4. Select a hair extension of the right color and length.

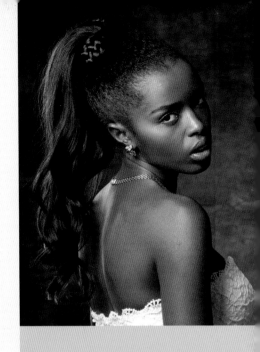

1

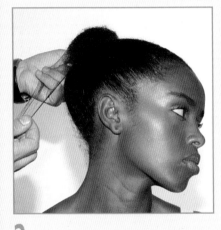

2

Enjoy long locks on your wedding day, even if your natural hair is quite short. In this design, two hair extensions are used to create a particularly long look.

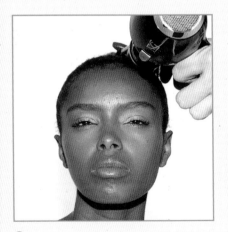

3

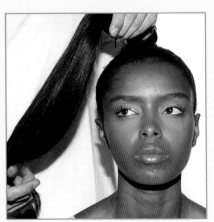

4

16

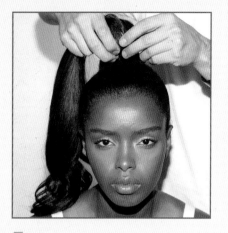

5

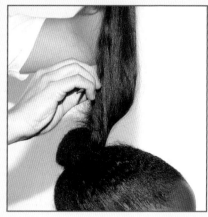

6

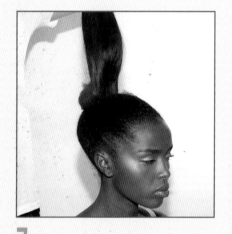

7

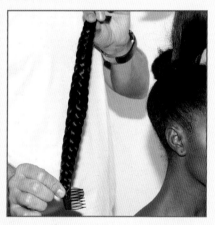

8

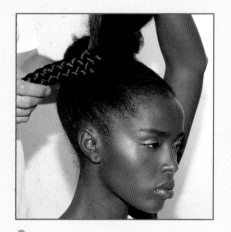

9

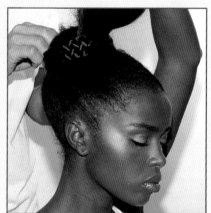

10

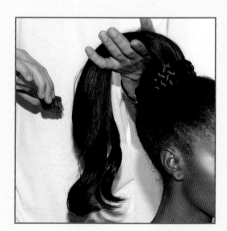

11

5. Affix the extension to the top of the ponytail with bobby pins, so that the extension covers the ponytail.

6. Backcomb the hair extension at the roots to create a thick, solid foundation for the hair that falls back.

7. Mist the backcombed base of the extension with holding spray. This will ensure that the additional volume lasts longer.

8. Select a braided hair extension (or braid an ordinary hair extension) that is the right color. Make sure it is long enough to wrap around the base of the ponytail.

9. Wrap the braided extensions over the front of the ponytail base and bring the ends around to the bottom of the ponytail.

10. Use bobby pins to secure the extension in place.

11. Gently brush the hair in the ponytail.

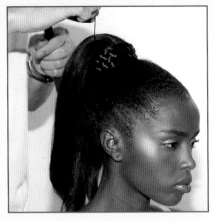

12

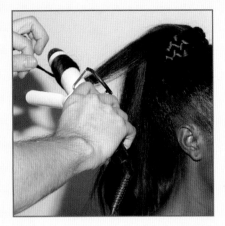

13

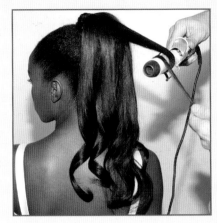

14

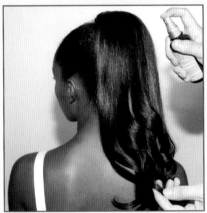

15

12. To secure the ponytail, insert bobby pins at the top of the ponytail into the area that was backcombed in step 6.

13. Make soft, open waves in the ponytail by curling sections of the ponytail with a medium-sized curling iron.

14. Make sure you curl the hair all the way to the ends.

15. Mist with holding spray to secure the hairstyle and add shine.

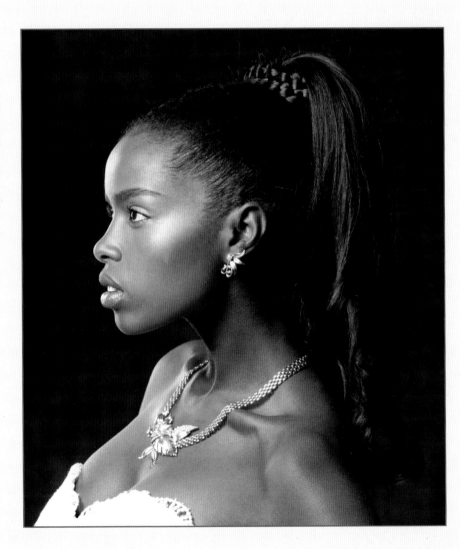

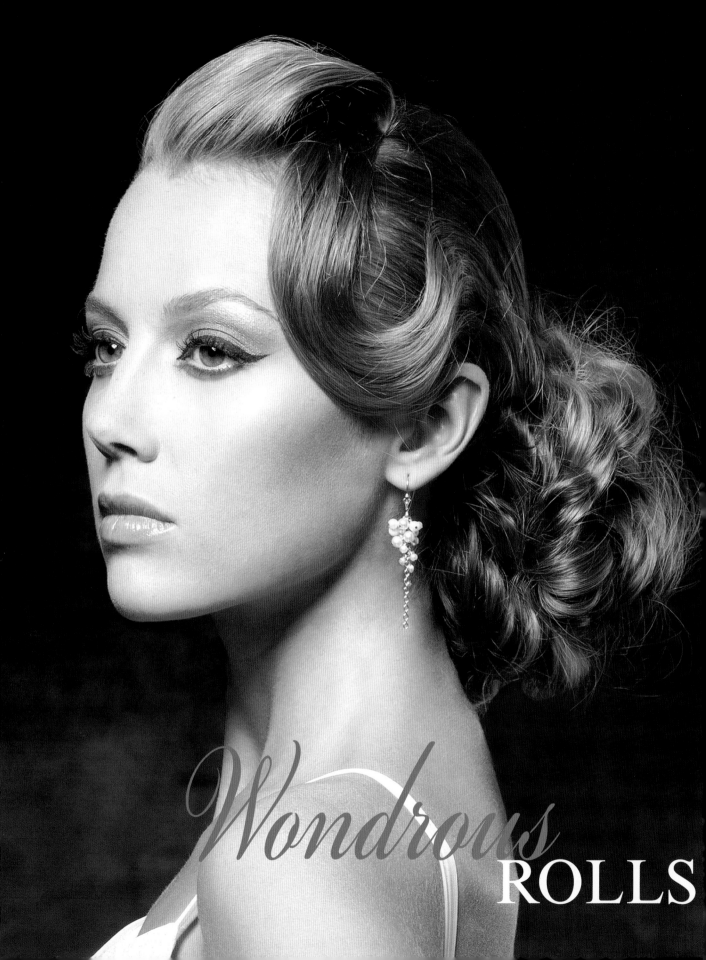

Wondrous ROLLS

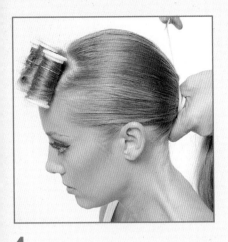

1

1. Wash and blow dry the hair. Separate the bangs from the rest of the hair and curl with hot rollers. Gather the rest of the hair at the back of the head in a low ponytail.

2. Affix a hair wrap around the base of the ponytail using bobby pins.

3. Roll a section of hair in the ponytail with a small curling iron. Hold the hair in the curling iron for about 10 seconds, then gently release. Repeat this technique to curl all the hair in the ponytail.

4. To increase the volume and create a more natural look, hold the ends of each curl and push back the hair with your fingers.

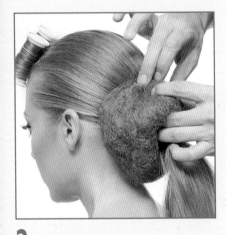

2

A rich collection of folded curls at the back and a seductive swirl at the front makes this hairstyle distinct, pretty, and perfect for every elegant bride.

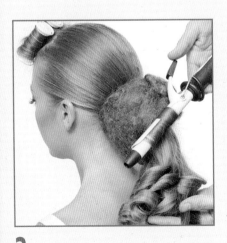

3

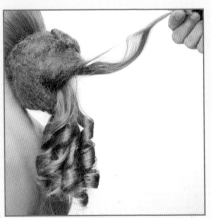

4

17

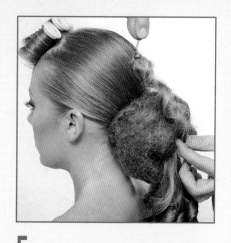

5

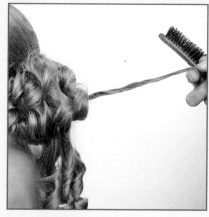

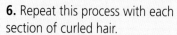

6

5. Roll the end of a curl into a bobby pin and then insert the bobby pin into the hair wrap, close to the scalp.

6. Repeat this process with each section of curled hair.

7. Make sure you don't pull out the curl when securing it to the hair wrap. Try to preserve a sense of movement and freedom in the curls.

8. After all the curls have been secured, use bobby pins to secure the curls to each other and over the hair wrap, covering it completely.

9. Release the bangs from the rollers.

10. Gently brush out the hair and backcomb it at the roots.

11. Draw the bangs backwards and twist them to increase the volume.

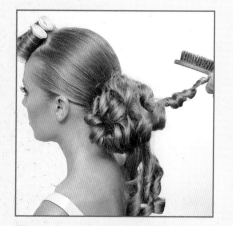

7

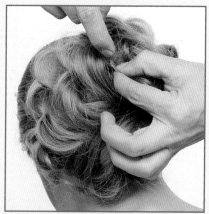

8

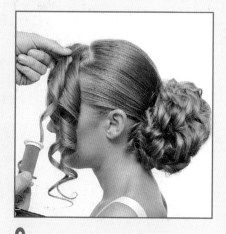

9

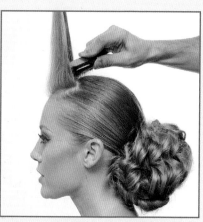

10

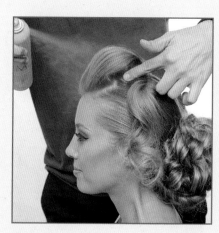

11

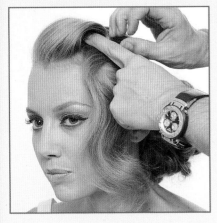

12

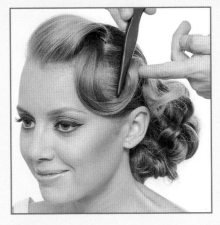

13

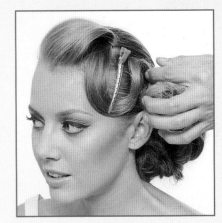

14

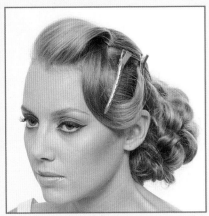

15

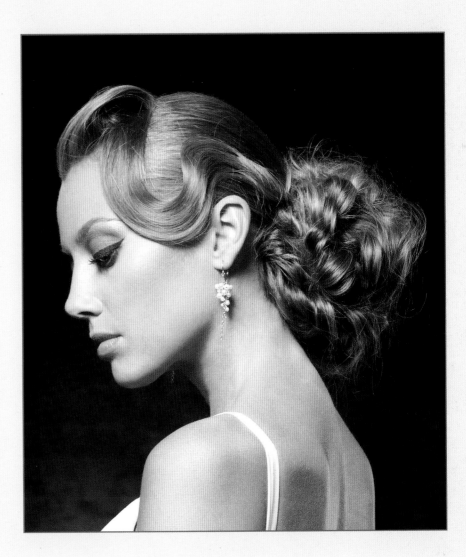

12. Secure the bangs by inserting a bobby pin close to the scalp.

13. Brush the bangs very gently and shape them into a soft wave.

14. Style the wave as you like and insert a hair clip to secure it in the desired position.

15. Insert another hair clip, if necessary, to hold the second part of the wave. When you're happy with the shape, mist with holding spray and wait for about 10 minutes. Gently remove the hair clips.

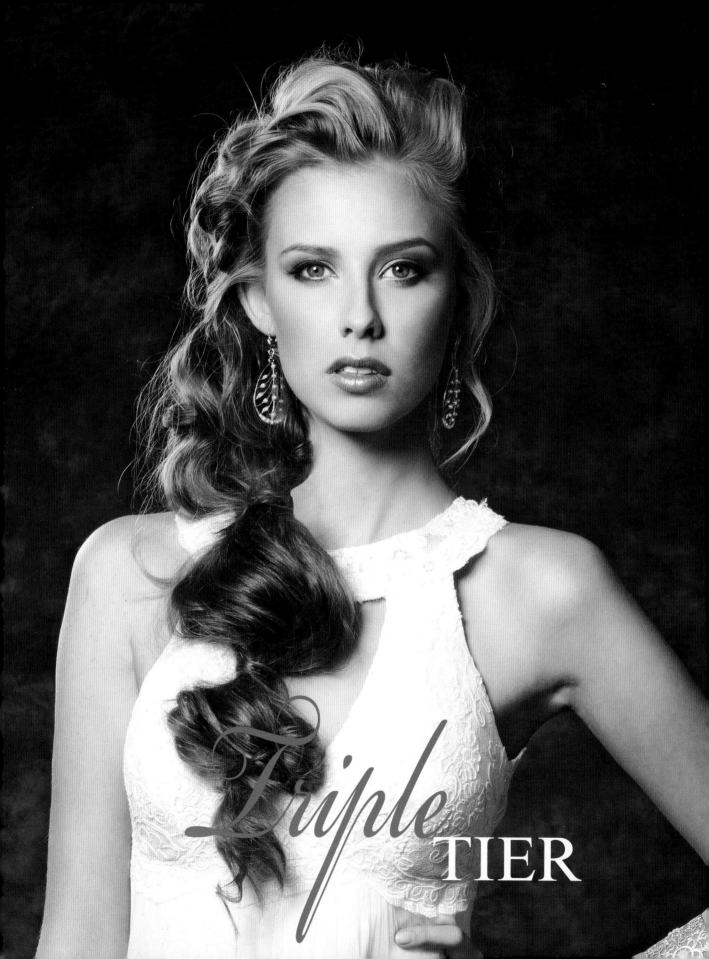

Triple TIER

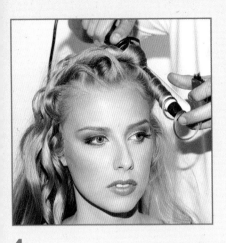

1. Wash and blow dry the hair. Roll the hair around the face into curls using a small curling iron.

2. Switch to a medium-sized curling iron and curl the hair at the crown of the head all the way to the roots. Make your way towards the back of the head, curling sections of hair as you go. Leave the hair curled until it cools.

3. Mist each curled section of hair with holding spray after curling to make the curls last.

4. Comb the hair at back of the head downwards, from the crown to the nape of the neck. Pin the hair behind the ear and mist with holding spray. This area is the base for the rest of the hairstyle.

1

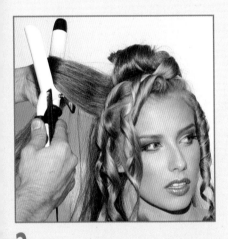

2

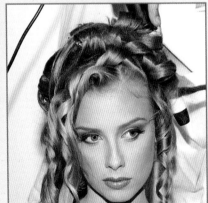

3

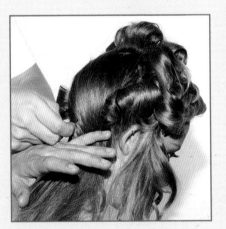

4

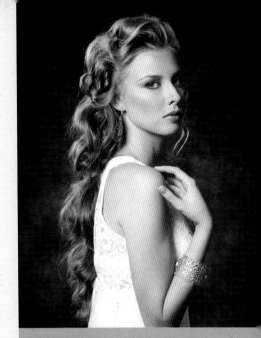

In this romantic design, the hair is collected in three swooping swirls at the front and twirled into a decorative back. Decorate with a few sprigs of baby's breath.

18

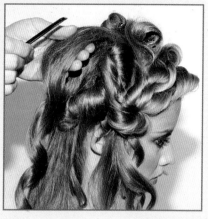

5

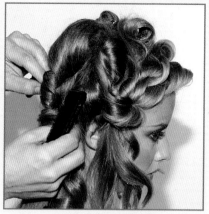

6

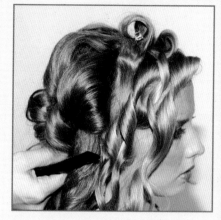

7

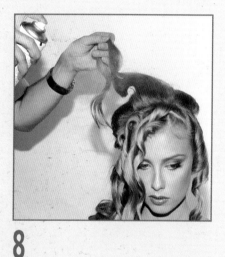

8

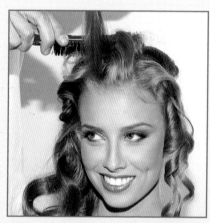

9

5. Gently release the curls, one at a time, making an effort to keep the hair wavy.

6. After releasing each curl, secure it near the base you formed in step 4.

7. To increase the volume and softness of each curl, backcomb each one gently only at the roots, and then softly brush it to create a gentle look.

8. Repeat this technique with each curl, all around the head. Mist with holding spray to secure the curls in place.

9. Make sure you treat each curl separately and carefully.

10. Continue drawing the curls gently backwards, collecting them at the nape of the neck, until you achieve the look you want.

11. Gather all the hair at one side of the head and hold it together with an elastic band.

12. Wrap another elastic band near the ends of the hair and a third elastic band between the first two.

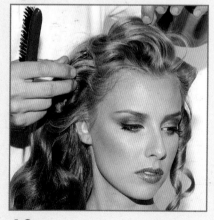

10

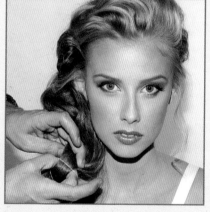

11

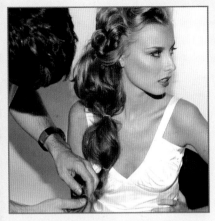

12

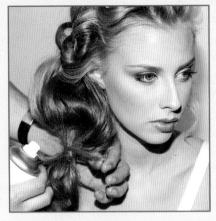

13

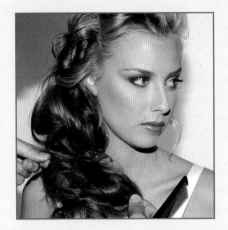

14

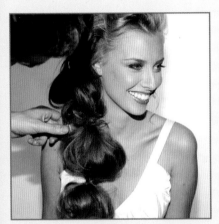

15

13. Draw out a small section of hair from the collected hair and wrap it around the top elastic band to conceal it. Repeat this process to conceal the other two elastic bands with sections of hair. Mist the wrapped hair with holding spray and secure with a bobby pin.

14. Gently draw out the hair between each elastic band with your fingers to add volume to each section.

15. Mist the hair with holding spray to keep the shape.

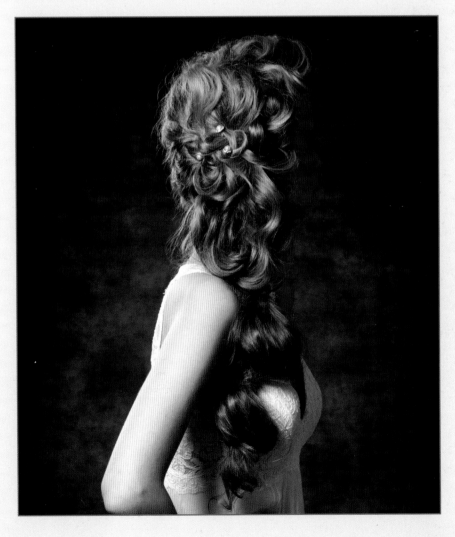

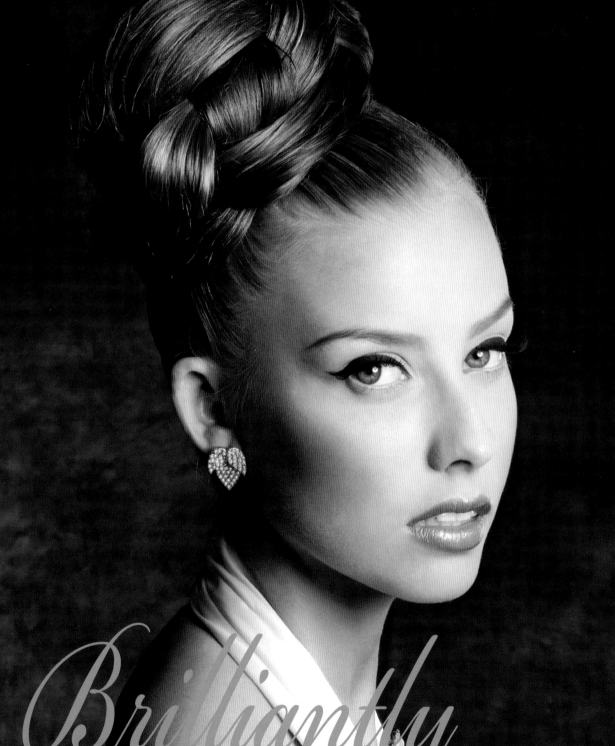

Brilliantly BRAIDED

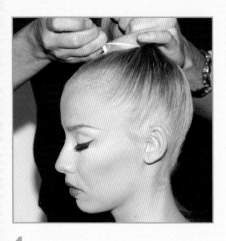

1. Wash and blow dry the hair. Brush the hair back and gather it in a high ponytail.

2. Divide the hair in the ponytail into four even sections. Place a bit of wax on your hand and rub some onto each section.

3. Grasp the rightmost section of hair from the ponytail, bring it over the 2nd section, and then under the 3rd section.

4. Now the rightmost section of hair is in your left hand.

1

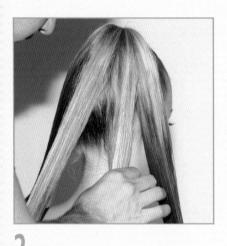

2

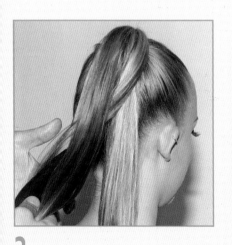

3

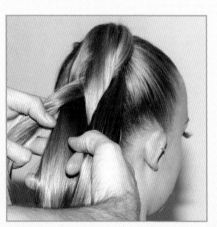

4

Increase the height of your hairstyle with a strategically placed hair wrap! In this design, the wrap is cleverly concealed with a 4-strand braid.

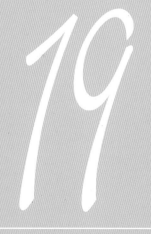

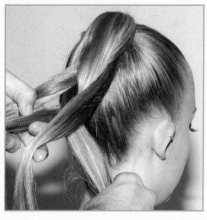

5

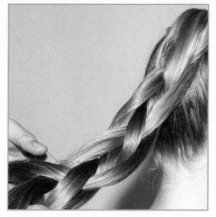

6

5. Grasp the section of hair that was originally on the left side (now it is 2nd from the left) and move it towards the right by bringing it over the adjacent section, and then under the last rightmost section. Now this section of hair is in your right hand.

6. Continue weaving the strands of hair in this manner, from right to left and then left to right, to create a 4-strand braid.

7. Secure the end of the braid with an elastic band and mist with a little holding spray.

8. Make sure the braid is secure, yet loose, with a relatively wide surface for covering the hair wrap.

9. Affix a hair wrap around the base of the ponytail with bobby pins.

10. Begin wrapping the braid around the hair wrap to conceal it.

11. Wrap the braid all around the hair wrap, securing it firmly with bobby pins.

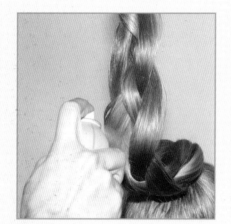

7

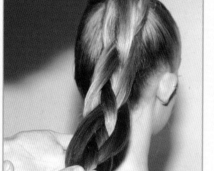

8

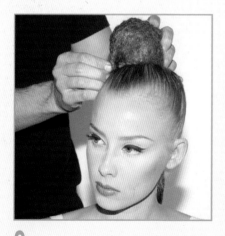

9

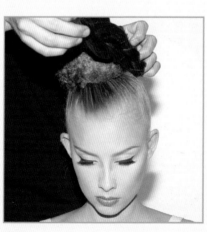

10

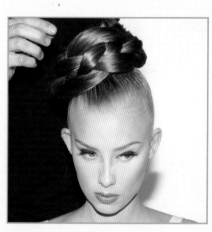

11

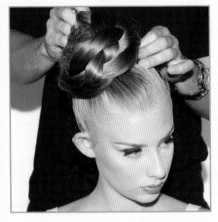

12

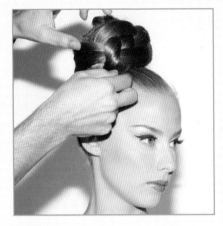

13

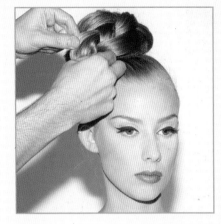

14

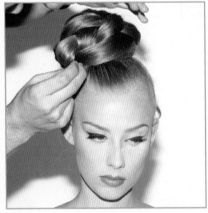

15

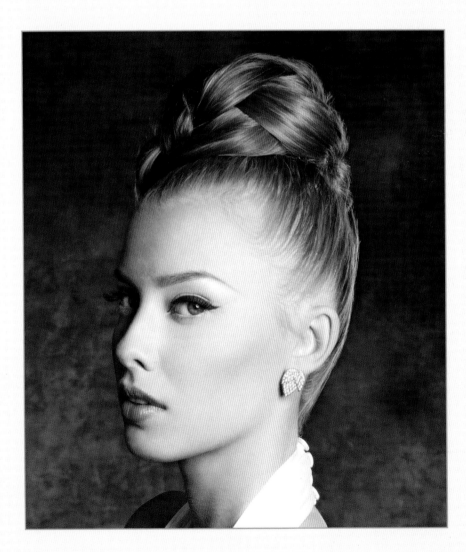

12. Insert bobby pins all around the braid, securing it to the scalp and the hair wrap.

13. Increase the surface area covered by the braid by gently massaging it with your fingers.

14. Gently draw out each section of hair until the hair wrap is fully covered.

15. Insert bobby pins throughout the braid, but don't open them fully to prevent them from being visible.

Creatively COILED

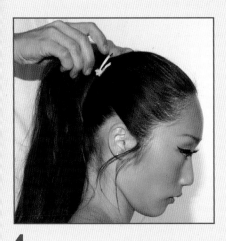

1. Wash and blow dry the hair. Brush the hair back and gather it in a high ponytail.

2. Divide the hair in the ponytail into two even sections.

3. Place a cylindrical sponge along the ends of one section of the ponytail and roll the hair downwards around the sponge, all the way to the roots.

4. When rolling the hair around the sponge, make it just as tight as when you roll hair around a roller. It's important to roll the hair tightly so that the shape of the sponge is preserved.

1

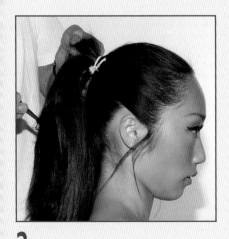

2

Look like a princess with this upswept double bun. Hair volume is increased in this design by wrapping the hair around cylindrical sponges!

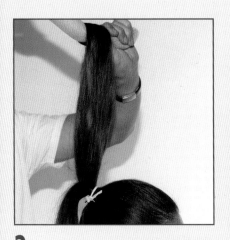

3

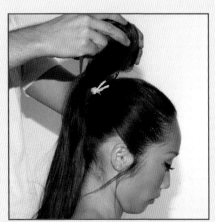

4

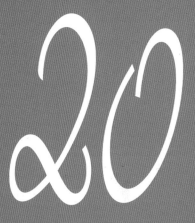

20

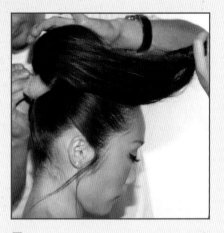

5

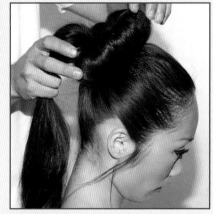

6

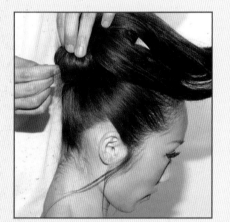

7

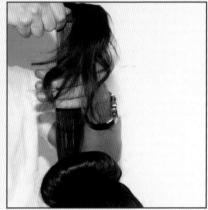

8

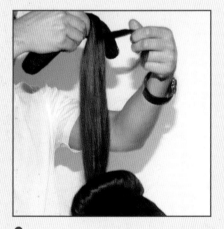

9

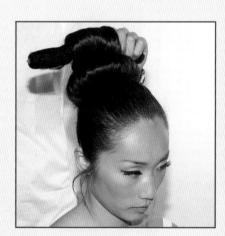

10

11

5. Wrap the sponge (now wrapped with hair) in a ring around the base of the ponytail and secure in place with bobby pins.

6. Using your fingers, gently massage the hair that's wrapped around the sponge in order to cover the entire area of the sponge.

7. To secure the wrapped hair, insert bobby pins all around it.

8. Brush out the other section of the ponytail.

9. Wrap this section of hair around another cylindrical sponge, from the ends of the hair all the way to the roots, just as you did with the first section of hair.

10. Wrap the hair tightly so that the shape of the sponge is preserved.

11. Continue rolling the hair until you reach the roots.

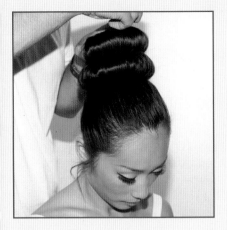

12

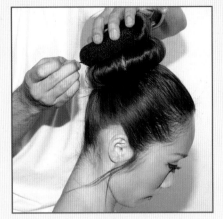

13

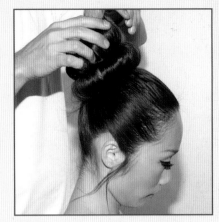

14

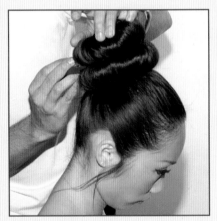

15

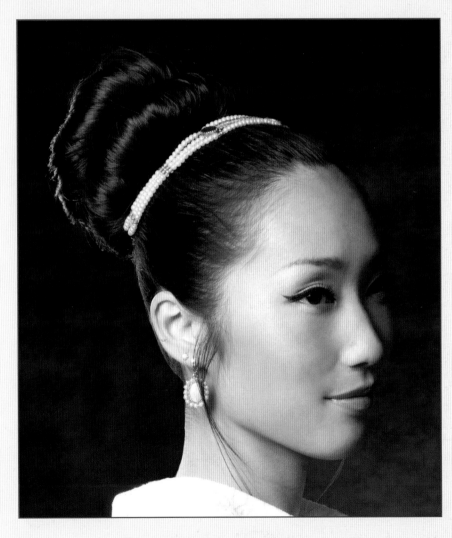

12. Form a ring with the wrapped sponge and place it on top of the first ring of hair. Make sure the ends of the wrapped sponge meet at the bottom of the head and then secure them together with bobby pins.

13. Secure the second ring on top of the first ring with bobby pins.

14. Massage the hair around the second ring, as you did with the first ring, until the entire sponge is concealed by hair.

15. Tuck in any stray ends of hair using a tail comb. Mist with holding spray.

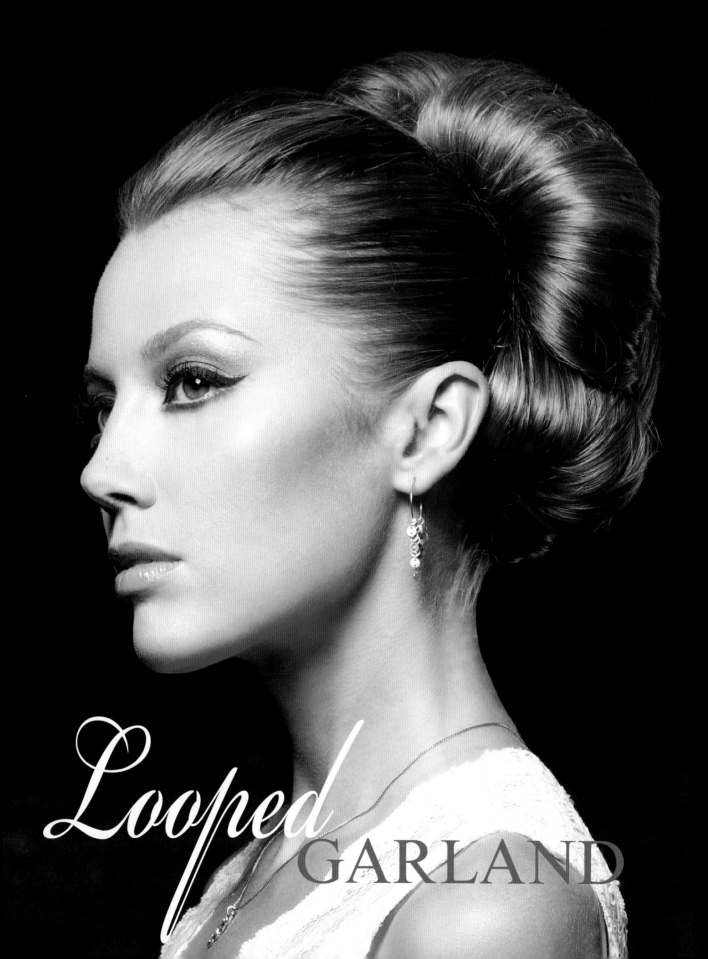

Looped GARLAND

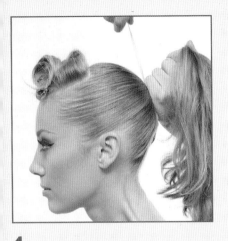

1 Wash and blow dry the hair. Separate the bangs from the rest of the hair. Hold the bangs with a hair clip and gather the rest of the hair in a high ponytail.

2. Release the bangs from the hair clip, mist with a little holding spray and brush backwards.

3. Draw the bangs to the back of the head, allow for a bit of volume at the top and secure just above the ponytail with bobby pins.

4. Divide the hair in the ponytail into five sections. Each section should be a different size. Fold each section towards the scalp and secure by inserting two bobby pins in an X shape.

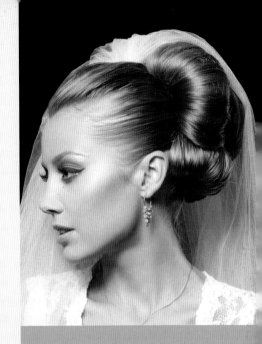

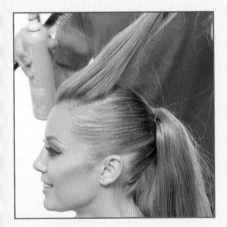

2

This beautiful hairstyle features several large rolls of hair gathered in an asymmetrical cluster at the back of the head. Dramatic and interesting.

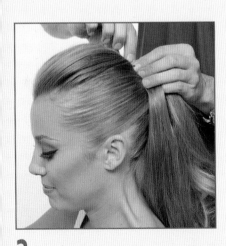

3

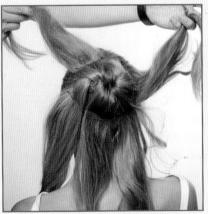

4

21

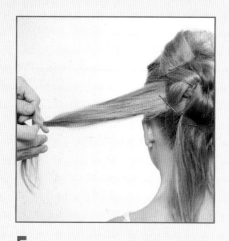

5

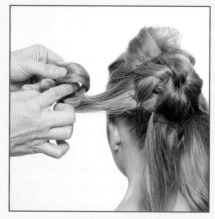

6

5. Brush out one section of hair and affix an elastic band near the end, about 8 inches from the scalp.

6. Backcomb the hair slightly above the elastic band and roll the hair upwards towards the scalp.

7. To secure the hair, insert a bobby pin through the elastic band and into the base of bobby pins that's already securing the hair to the scalp. To make it even more secure, you could insert additional bobby pins on either side of the rolled hair.

8. Repeat this technique with another section of hair. Roll the hair in a different direction to create an interesting arrangement.

9. When securing each rolled section of hair, make sure it touches the adjacent section.

10. Shift the rolled sections of hair, if necessary, so that all of them are connected.

11. Roll another section of hair at the crown of the head.

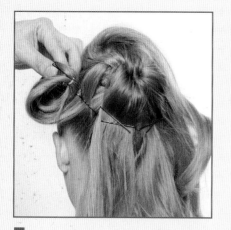

7

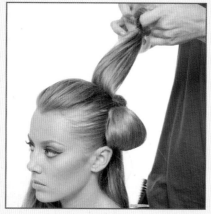

8

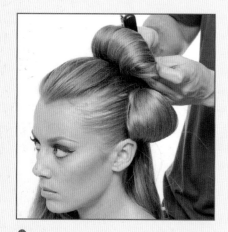

9

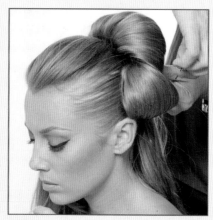

10

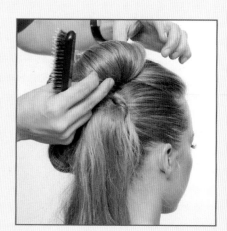

11

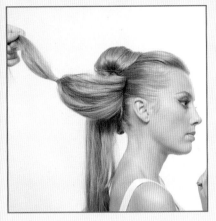

12

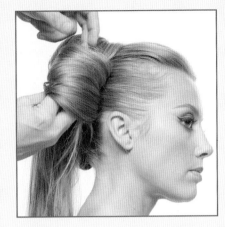

13

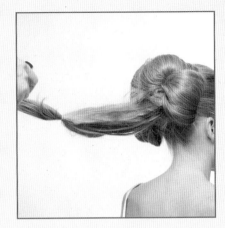

14

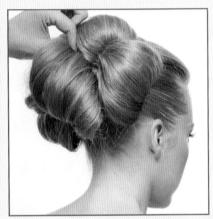

15

12. Make sure each section is positioned in a different manner.

13. To increase the volume of the hairstyle, make sure that the rolls of hair that you affix extend beyond the frame of the face.

14. In the same manner, continue rolling and securing the sections of hair at the back of the head.

15. Roll up the last section of hair and pin it just above the base of the ponytail. Mist with holding spray to secure it.

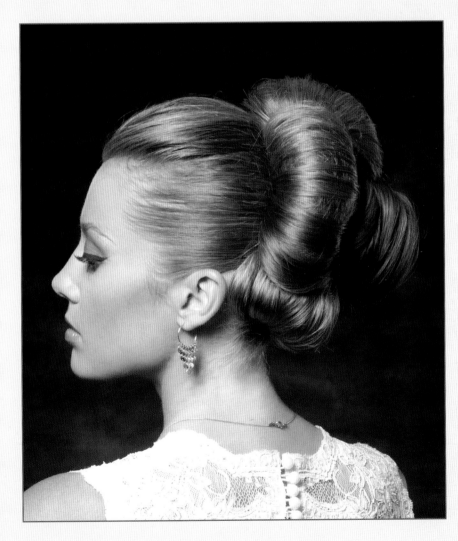

The Princess BRIDE

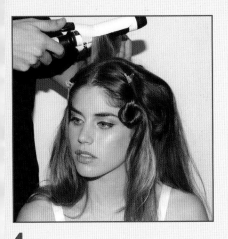

1

1. Wash and blow dry the hair. Divide the hair into front and back sections by making a part over the crown of the head, from one ear to the other. Mist a section of hair from the back section of the hair with holding spray and then curl with a medium-sized curling iron.

2. Hold the hair in the curling iron for about 15 seconds and then gently release to create a solid curl. Secure the curl with a hair clip.

3. Repeat this process to curl all the hair at the back of the head. Let the curls set for about 10 minutes.

4. Move to the front section of hair and grasp two small sections of hair, each about 1 inch wide, above one ear. Rub a bit of wax onto each section of hair and twist the sections until they each resemble a rope.

5. Draw the lower section of hair upwards and the higher section of hair downwards to form an X shape.

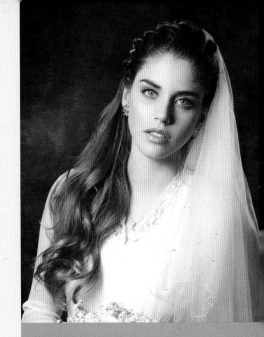

This gorgeous design features a twisted rope of hair wrapped over the top of the head like a hair band. Distinctive, pretty, and fit for a princess!

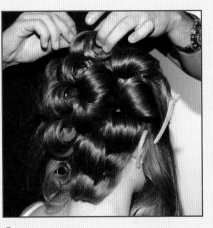

2

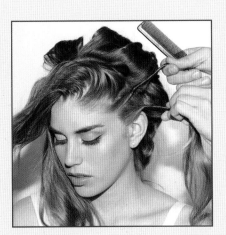

3

4

22

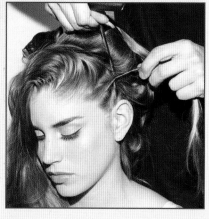

5

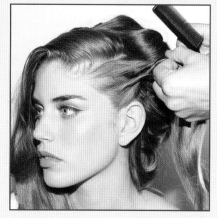

6

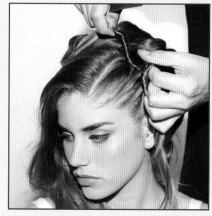

7

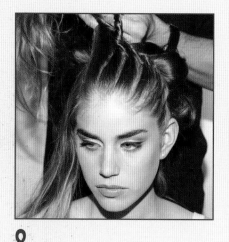

8

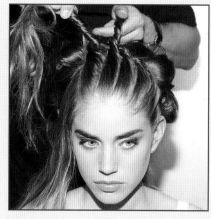

9

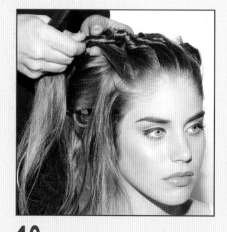

10

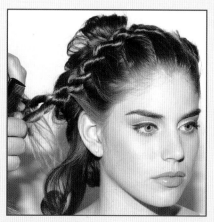

11

6. Move upwards along this side of the head and grasp another 1-inch section of hair. Twist this section together with the lower section of hair (which you drew upwards when making the X) to form a single twisted section of hair.

7. Bring the section of hair now closest to the ear upwards and under the top section of hair. Draw out another 1-inch section of hair and twist it together with this section.

8. Repeat this technique to incorporate 1-inch sections of hair all over the front of the head. Every time you incorporate another section of hair, make sure it is rolled into a rope with the section of hair that is under it, in order to create twisted trails of hair all around the face.

9. As you make your way from one ear to the other, the rope of hair that acts as a head band becomes thicker.

10. Make sure you stand behind the bride as you twist the hair, since you want to draw each section of hair backwards with the same degree of tightness.

11. As each section of hair is added, it must be twisted tightly and in the same direction as the previous twist.

12. Continue twisting each section of hair into a rope. Continue twisting the

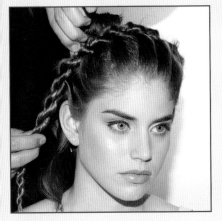

12

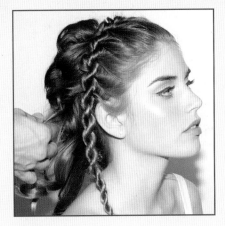

13

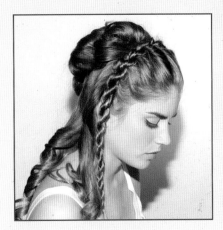

14

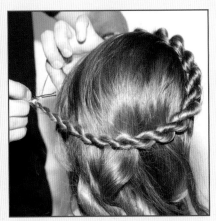

15

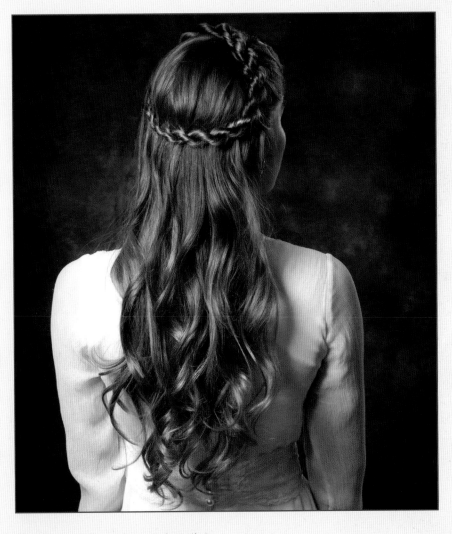

ropes together, even after you have finished incorporating new sections of hair. Twist the two sections around each other all the way to the end of the hair and then secure with an elastic band. Gently pull out strands of hair from the twisted rope to soften the look and increase the volume.

13. Gently release the hair clips from the curls at the back of the head.

14. Using your fingers, gently release the curls until the hair is loose and wavy.

15. Draw the twisted rope of hair around the back of the head like a crown. If the hair is long enough, secure the end by pinning it at the front of the head, just above the ear where the twisted roll started. Mist with holding spray to secure it.

Wrapped WAVES

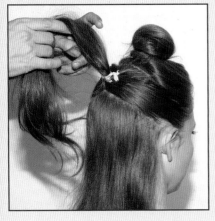

1. Wash and blow dry the hair. Divide the hair into three sections: a front section that includes the bangs; a middle section that extends from behind the bangs to above the ears; and a back section that includes the hair at the back of the head. Secure the front and middle sections with elastic bands.

2. Roll the middle section of hair with a large curling iron and secure with a hair clip. Repeat to curl the back section into a large curl.

3. Bring the hair at the front of the head forwards and backcomb at the roots.

4. Draw the hair backwards and gently brush the side of the hair that is now visible to achieve a neat look. Mist the hair with a little holding spray.

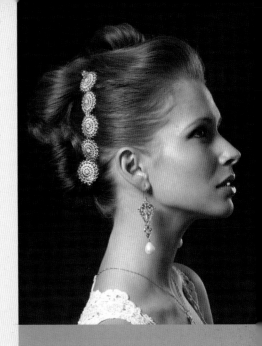

Seemingly simple from the front, this design features an opulent back with shapely, thick waves of hair. Dress it up with a decorative hair clip.

1

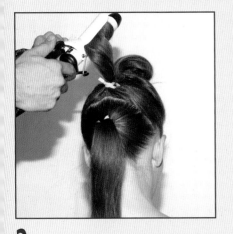

2

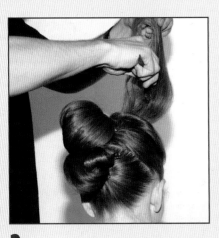

3

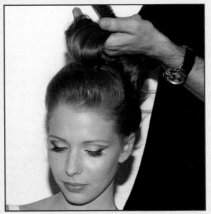

4

23

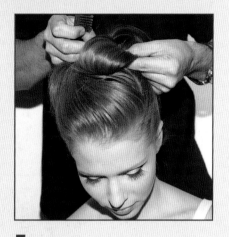

5

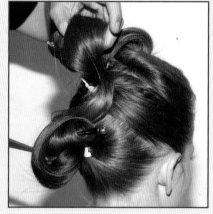

6

5. Secure the hair at the back of the head with a bobby pin.

6. Using your fingers or a tail comb, wrap the ends of this section of hair around the bases of the other two ponytails.

7. Bring the hair from the ponytail at the middle of the head upwards and wrap it around the hair from the front of the head. Bring the hair in this ponytail back towards the back of the head and secure with a hair clip.

8. Brush the hair in the opposite direction and secure with a little holding spray.

9. Roll the ponytail at the bottom of the head around the base of the middle ponytail.

10. Wrap this hair upwards, form a loop at the end, and secure beside the middle ponytail using a hair clip.

11. Note how three separate sections of hair were twisted together to create a single, sculpted look.

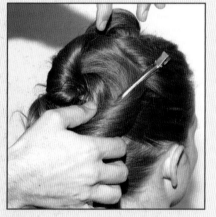

7

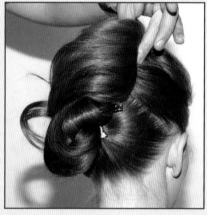

8

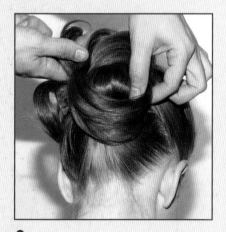

9

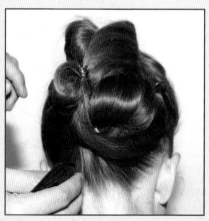

10

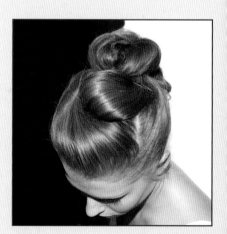

11

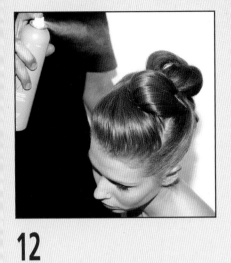

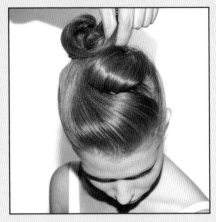

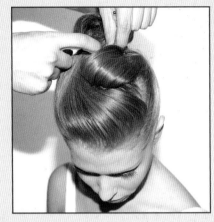

12

13

14

12. Mist the entire hairstyle with holding spray and dry with a diffuser.

13. Once the hair is secure, gently release the hairclips that are holding the design in place.

14. Secure the hairstyle for the evening by inserting bobby pins throughout the hairstyle.

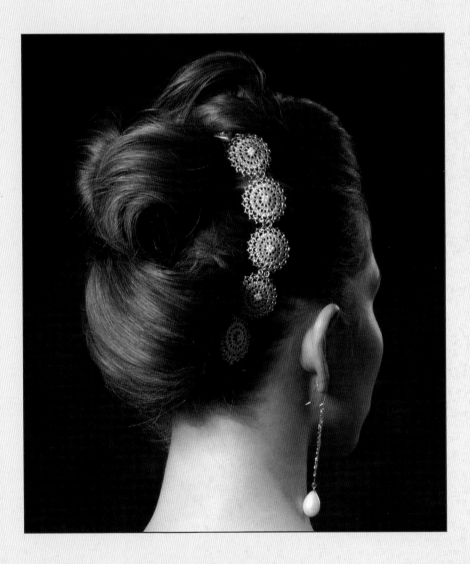

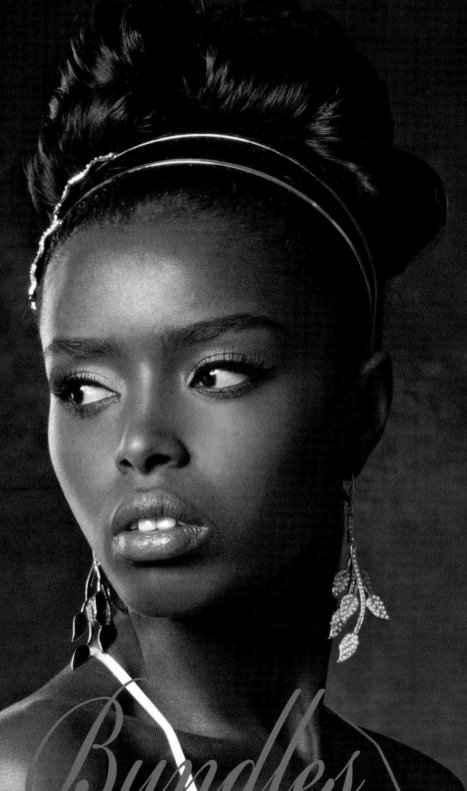

Bundles OF JOY

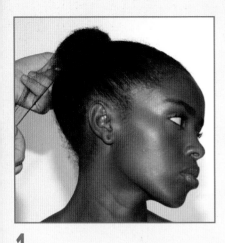

1

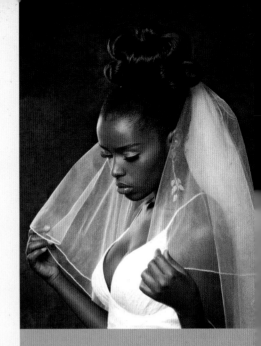

1. Wash and blow dry the hair. Brush the hair back and gather it in a high ponytail. Select a hairnet that matches the color of the hair and wrap it around the ponytail.

2. Select a hair extension that matches the color of the hair and affix it to the ponytail with bobby pins.

3. Divide the extension into several sections and mist each section with holding spray. Wrap each section around a hot roller. Be sure to roll the entire length of the extension around each roller.

4. Keep the hair in rollers for about 10 minutes, until completely cool.

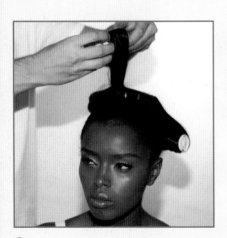

2

Be extravagant by curling several extensions into rich rolled curls. The overall look is both playful and sophisticated.

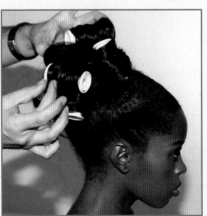

3

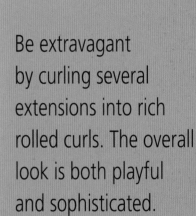

4

24

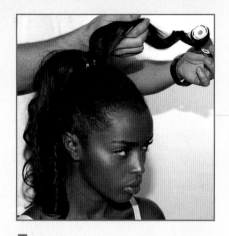

5

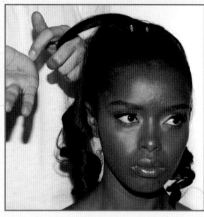

6

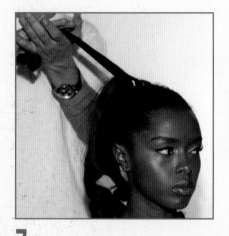

7

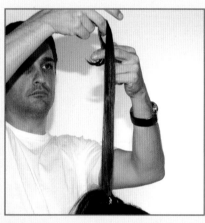

8

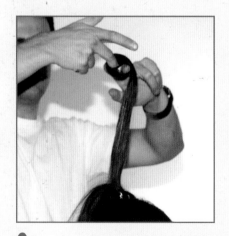

9

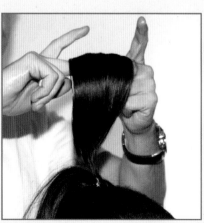

10

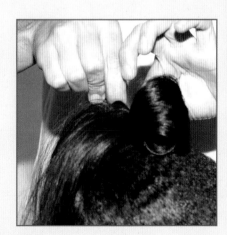

11

5. Gently release the rollers.

6. Spread a bit of wax on your hand and rub it along each curl for a clean, shiny look.

7. Make sure you apply the wax all the way to the end of the hair to keep the entire curl unified.

8. Draw one curled section of hair upwards and roll the end.

9. Using both hands, roll the hair into a hollow curl by holding the hair with one hand and using the fingers of the other hand to roll it.

10. Continue rolling the hair towards the roots until you achieve a loop that is just the right size.

11. Secure the loop to the scalp by inserting a pin along the length of the loop, close to the scalp. Mist the loop with holding spray to secure it.

12. Repeat this technique with the other curls.

13. Spray each rolled section of hair with holding spray after securing it to the scalp in order to retain the shape.

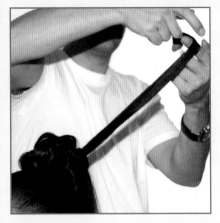

12

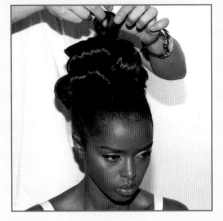

13

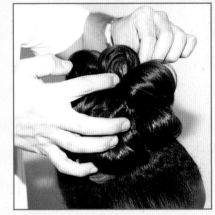

14

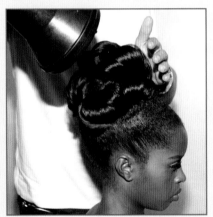

15

14. Note that not all the loops will be pinned to the scalp. After the first batch of loops has been pinned, the loops that follow are pinned to previous loops (rather than to the scalp).

15. When all the loops are in place, mist the entire hairstyle with holding spray. Drying with a diffuser helps to hold the hairstyle perfectly in place.

16. To place the veil, insert the comb directly below the looped area of the hairstyle. When removing the veil, make sure you pull out the comb in the exact opposite direction.

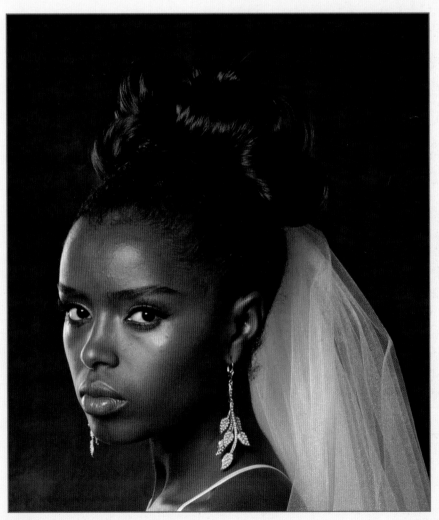

16

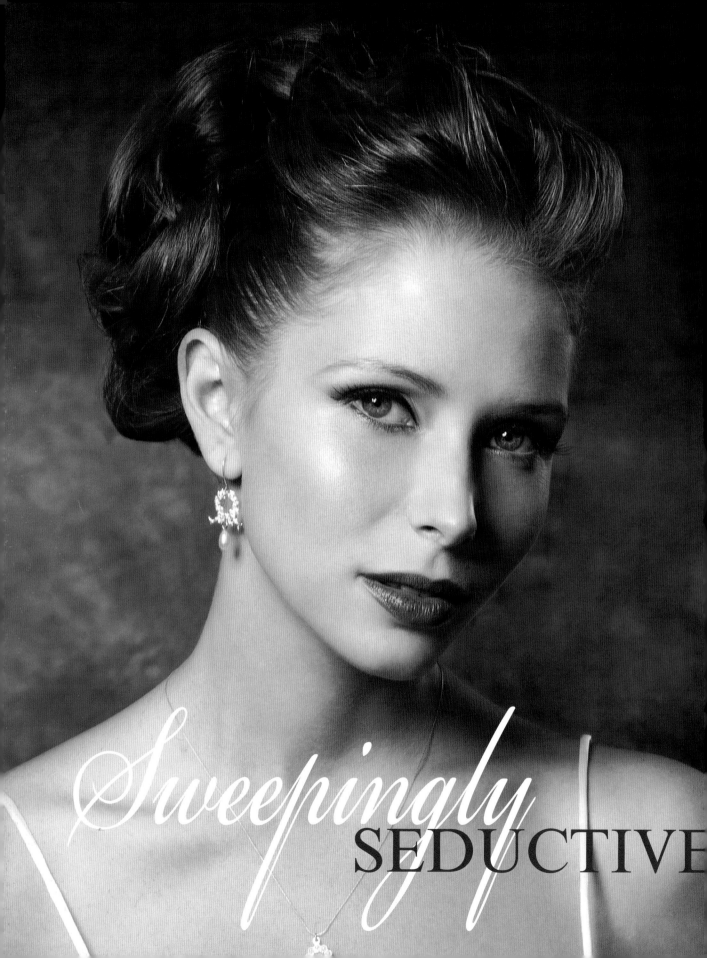

Sweepingly SEDUCTIVE

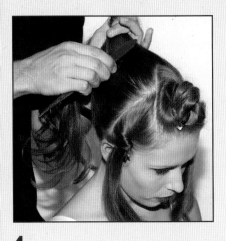

1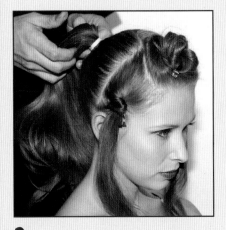

2

1. Wash and blow dry the hair. Divide it into four sections: a triangular section at the bangs; two small sections that extend from the crown of the head over each ear; and one section at the back of the head.

2. Gather the hair at the back of the head in a low ponytail.

3. Draw the hair over one ear towards the back of the head. Make sure the hair is brushed flat and close to the scalp and then wrap it tightly around the base of the ponytail. Secure with bobby pins. Repeat this technique with the hair over the other ear as well.

4. Mist the hair at the front of the head with holding spray and then curl using a small curling iron.

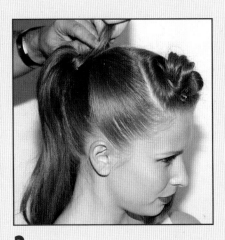

3

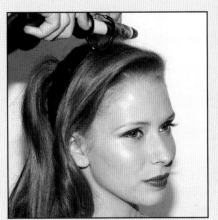

4

Keep the neck beautifully bare with this romantic hairstyle. It features soft curls that are folded and then tucked at the back of the head.

25

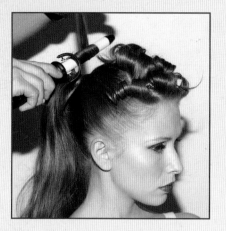

5

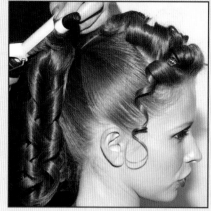

6

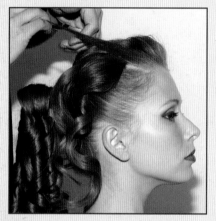

7

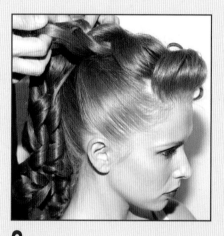

8

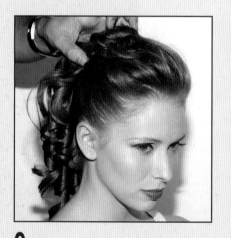

9

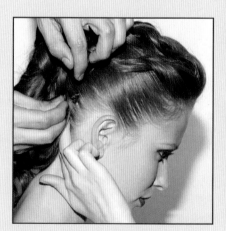

10

11

5. Use the same curling iron to curl the hair in the ponytail.

6. Hold each section in the curling iron for about 10 seconds before releasing it to ensure a firm curl.

7. Spread a little wax on your hand and rub the wax along the length of each curl to give it a soft, smooth look.

8. Once all the curls have been treated with wax, draw the curls from the front of the head towards the back in a single, thick group.

9. Secure these curls at the base of the ponytail with bobby pins.

10. Secure each curled section of hair separately by twisting the end of the curl and securing it with a bobby pin.

11. Insert the closed side of the pin through the hair that is drawn into the ponytail.

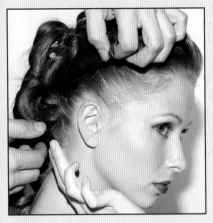

12

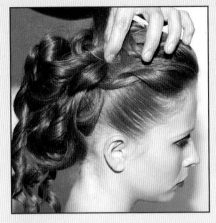

13

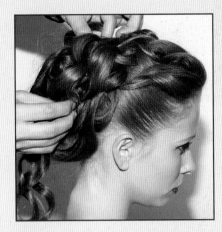

14

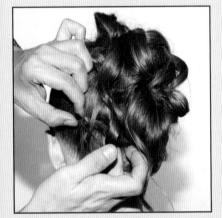

15

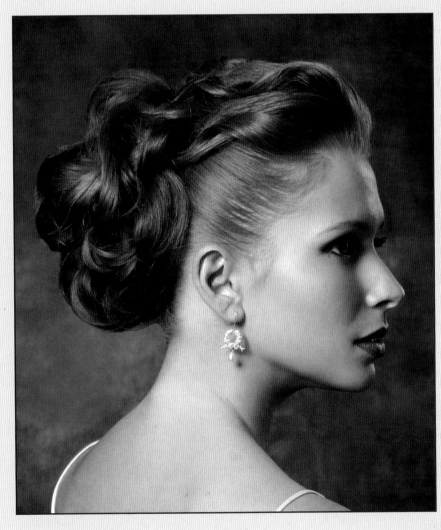

12. Imagine you are inserting the bobby pin into the hair in the same way as you would insert a sewing needle into fabric. The end of the bobby pin should be secured inside the ponytail.

13. Repeat this technique with all the curled sections of hair, pinning them to the hair in the ponytail.

14. Secure a different section of hair each time.

15. Make sure that the curls are well-coated with wax before you begin pinning them, since this makes it easier to handle the curls. Mist with holding spray.

Very VICTORIAN

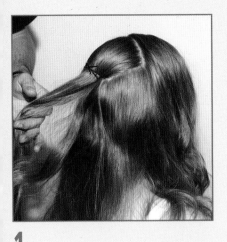

1

1. Wash and blow dry the hair. Mark off a section of hair at the crown of the head and backcomb it at the roots. Brush the hair backwards and secure it by inserting bobby pins in an X shape.

2. Wrap an elastic band around the gathered hair, about 5 inches from the bobby pins, and backcomb the ends (below the elastic band) to increase volume.

3. Roll the gathered hair upwards towards the scalp.

4. Secure the elastic band to the scalp with bobby pins to create a roll of hair.

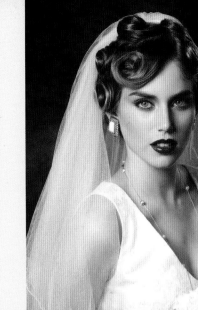

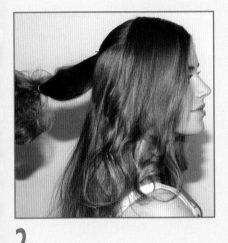

2

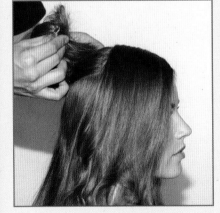

3

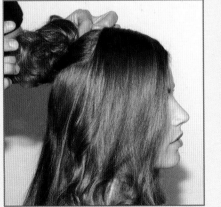

4

This daring design is sure to impress every guest at your wedding. It features dozens of twisted curls arranged all over the head. Exquisite and striking!

26

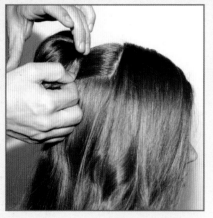

5

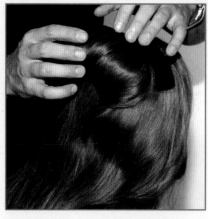

6

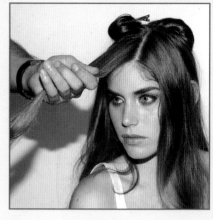

7

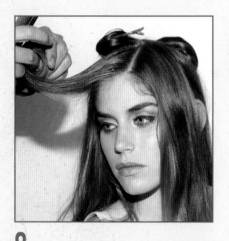

8

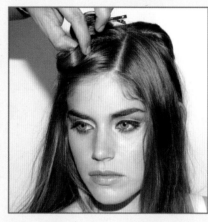

9

5. Tuck the backcombed ends of the hair into the roll.

6. Shift the rolled hair towards the scalp and secure it with bobby pins.

7. Make a part in the hair at the front of the head and grasp a 2-inch section of hair on one side of the part. Mist the hair with a little holding spray.

8. Roll this section of hair around your fingers, from the end of the hair towards the roots, to form a coil.

9. Secure the coiled hair to the scalp with a hair clip.

10. Mist the hair with holding spray and let it dry.

11. Repeat this process to coil all the hair at the front of the head, rolling 2-inch sections of hair into coils and securing them with bobby pins.

12. Spray each section of hair with holding spray before rolling it, in order to make the hairstyle last longer.

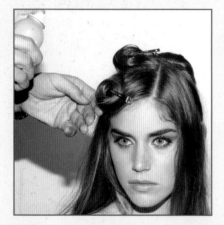

10

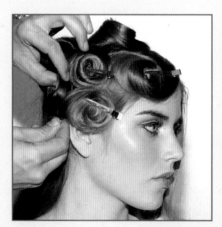

11

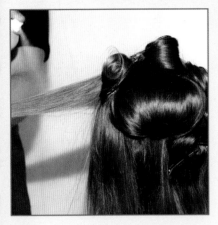

12

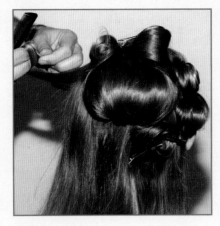

13

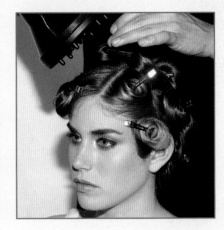

14

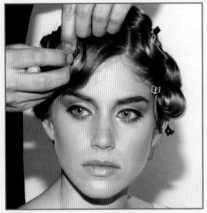

15

13. After rolling the hair around your finger and securing it to the scalp, mist each section of hair with holding spray.

14. Using a diffuser, heat the hair for about 5 minutes and then let it cool for about 10 minutes.

15. Once the hair has set, gently remove the hair clips from each roll of hair and replace them with bobby pins. Make sure you insert the bobby pins in an X shape so that they are really secure and then conceal the pins with the hair.

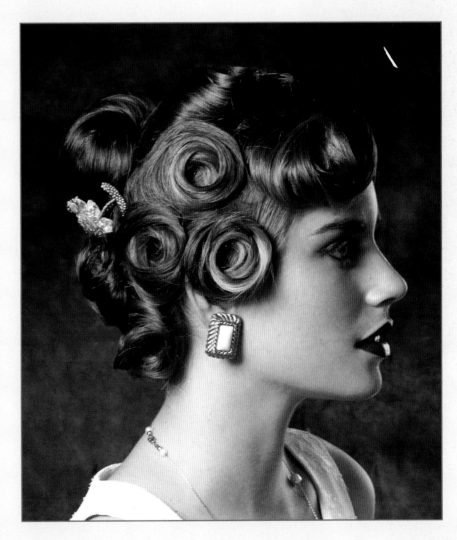

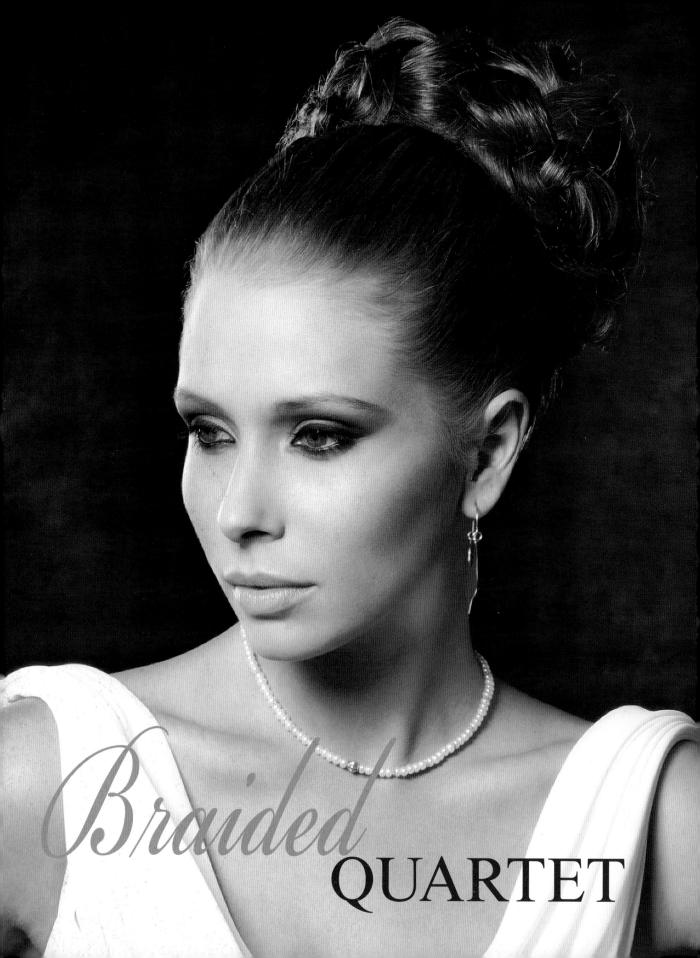

Braided QUARTET

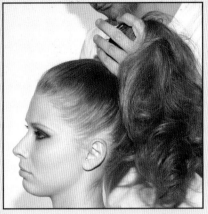

1. Wash and blow dry the hair. Brush the hair back and gather it in a high ponytail.

2. When wrapping the elastic band around the ponytail, make sure it is quite tight.

3. Affix a long hair wrap around the top of the ponytail to add volume. Hold the hair wrap in place with bobby pins.

4. Bring the ends of the hair wrap around to the bottom of the ponytail and hold in place with bobby pins. Make sure the ponytail hangs freely over the extension.

1

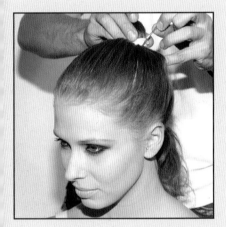

2

Make the most of your straight hair with this smooth design. Increase the volume by affixing a hair wrap at the back and wrapping it with simple braids.

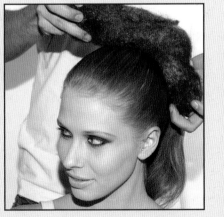

3

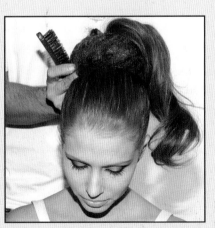

4

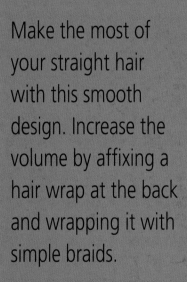

27

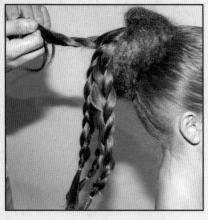

5

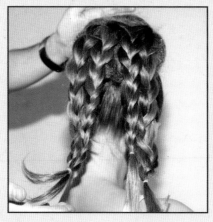

6

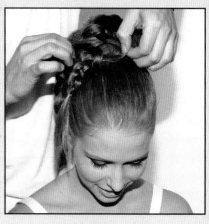

7

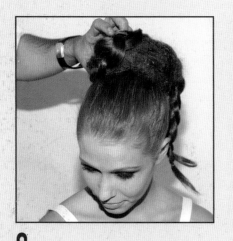

8

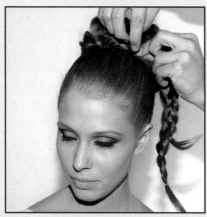

9

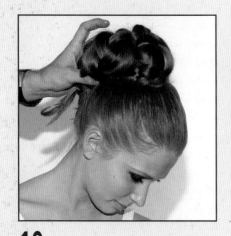

10

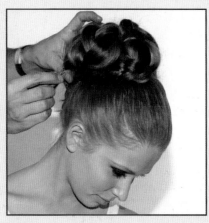

11

5. Divide the hair in the ponytail into four equal sections and separate each section into three even sections. Rub a bit of wax onto each of these sections and then braid them. Secure the bottom of each braid with an elastic band.

6. Repeat this technique to form braids in each of the four sections.

7. Wrap the braids around the hair wrap in an effort to conceal the wrap.

8. Open the braids gently with your fingers so that the natural hair covers the entire area of the wrap.

9. After all the braids have been pinned, massage them gently with your fingers to loosen them even more and increase their coverage of the hair wrap.

10. Repeat this process at the back of the head as well.

11. The size of each braid will be a bit different now, resulting in an interesting texture and look.

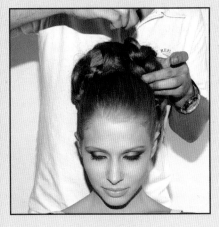

12

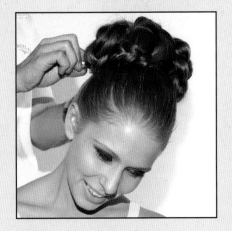

13

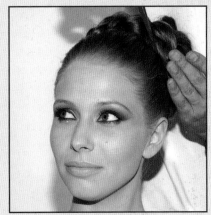

14

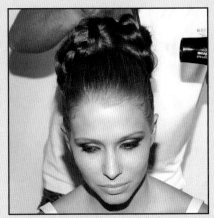

15

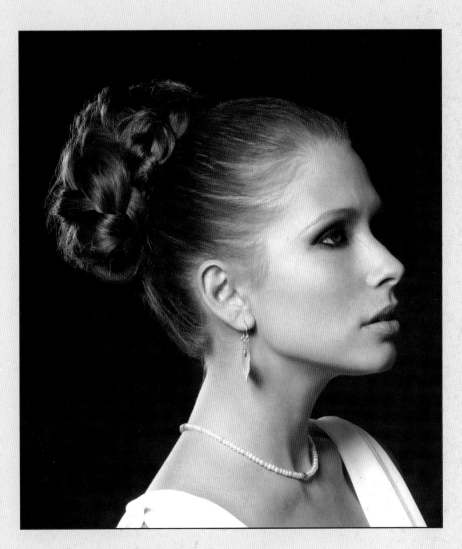

12. Use bobby pins to connect the braids to each other and ensure complete coverage of the hair wrap.

13. Repeat this technique all around the hair until it looks just right.

14. Use a tail comb to brush the hair back smoothly and tuck in the loose hair ends.

15. Mist the entire hairstyle with holding spray and blow dry for a classic, clean finish.

Glamour GIRL

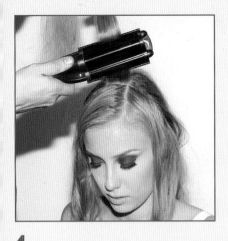

1. Wash and blow dry the hair. Divide the hair into front and back sections with a part that extends over the crown of the head. Make a side part in the front section of hair. Grasp a 2-inch section of hair immediately behind the crown of the head and crimp with a wave iron.

2. Mist each section of hair with holding spray before crimping it with the wave iron.

3. Crimp all the hair in the back section of the hair, all the way to the ends.

4. Collect some of the crimped hair in a high ponytail at the back of the head.

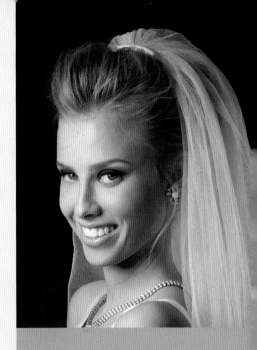

1

2

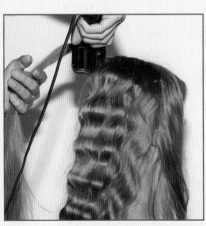

This upswept design adds height and elegance. The neck is left enticingly bare and the loose strands of hair are enchanting.

3

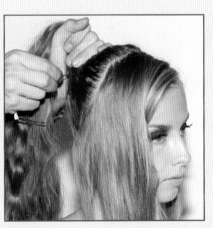

4

28

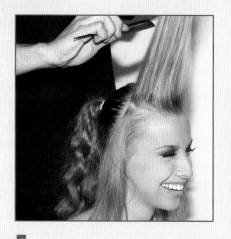

5

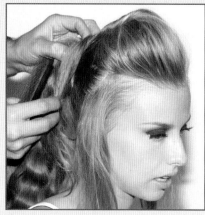

6

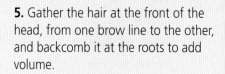

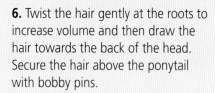

5. Gather the hair at the front of the head, from one brow line to the other, and backcomb it at the roots to add volume.

6. Twist the hair gently at the roots to increase volume and then draw the hair towards the back of the head. Secure the hair above the ponytail with bobby pins.

7. Brush the hair at the sides of the head upwards and towards the back. Secure at the base of the ponytail with bobby pins.

8. Divide the hair in the ponytail into two sections and twist each section around itself.

9. Roll the two twisted sections of hair together, like a rope. Make sure the twisted hair remains loose and interesting.

10. Hold the end of the twisted rope of hair and draw out strands of hair all along the length of it to make the texture even more interesting.

11. Secure the end of the hair with an elastic band.

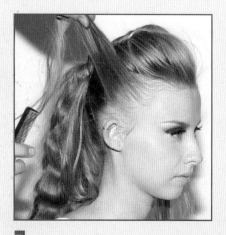

7

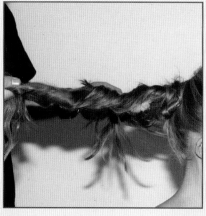

8

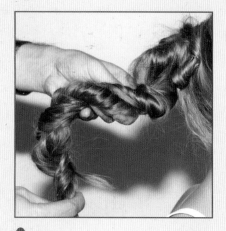

9

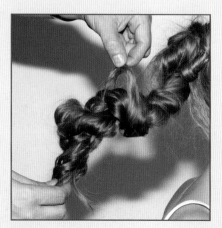

10

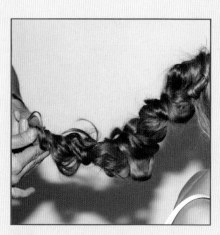

11

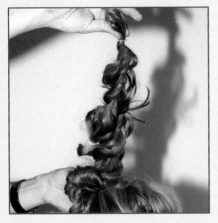

12

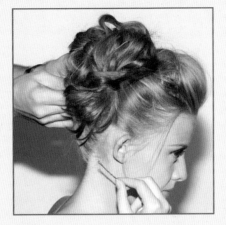

13

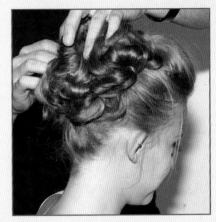

14

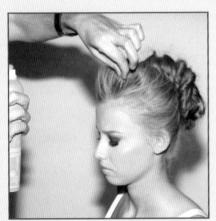

15

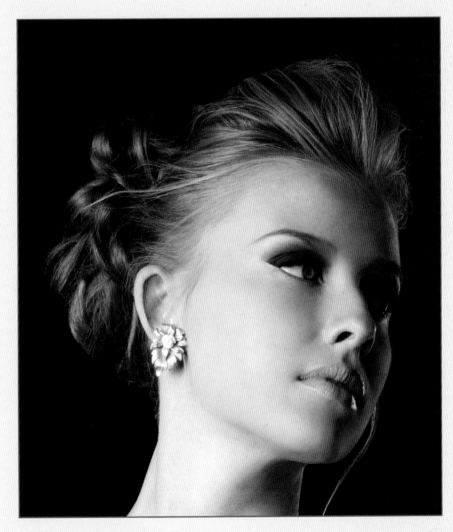

12. Roll the twisted rope of hair around the base of the ponytail.

13. Make sure you don't twist the hair too tightly, since that could diminish the interesting texture you've created.

14. Secure the rolled and twisted hair to the scalp using as many bobby pins as necessary.

15. Mist the hairstyle with holding spray to secure it. Draw out a few strands around the face to soften the style and frame the face.

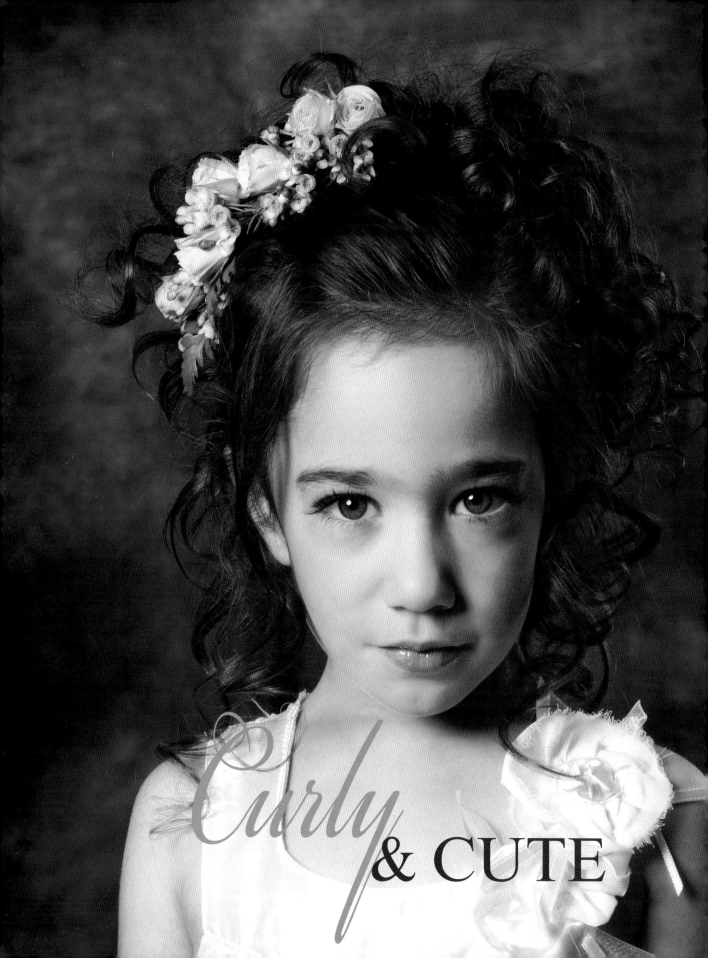

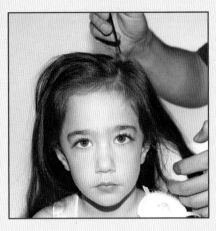

1. Wash and blow dry the hair.

2. Divide the hair into front and back sections by making a part over the top of the head and towards the back, from one ear to the other.

3. Collect the hair at the back of the head in a high ponytail.

4. Curl the hair framing the face using a small curling iron.

1

2

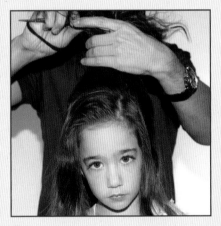

This playful style is perfect for a young bridesmaid. To make the bridesmaid feel even more special, add a few real flowers.

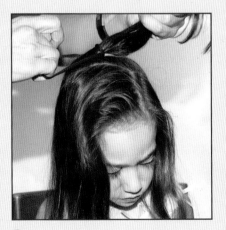

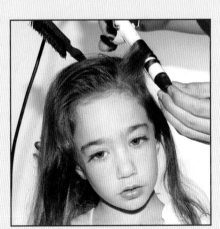

3

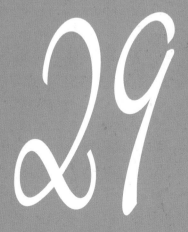

4

29

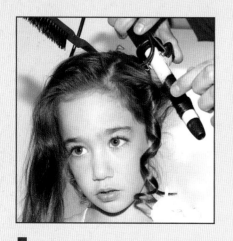

5

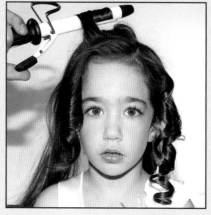

6

5. To help secure the curl, mist each section of hair with holding spray before curling it.

6. Let each curl set for about 10 seconds before gently releasing the hair from the curling iron.

7. When all the hair at the front of the head has been curled, move to the back of the head and continue curling sections of hair.

8. Repeat this technique all around the head.

9. Loosen the curls gently with your fingers to create a soft, wavy look.

10. Gently draw the hair at the front of the head towards the back and gather it in a high ponytail.

11. Make sure you leave the waves in the hair as you draw each section backwards to make the ponytail.

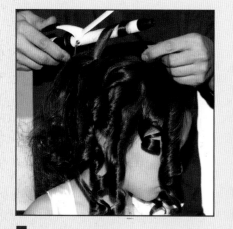

7

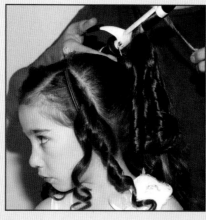

8

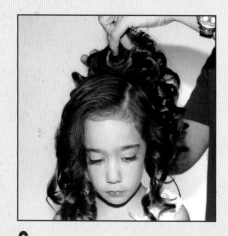

9

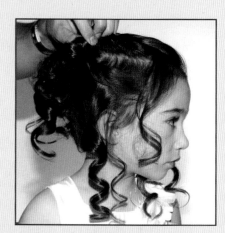

10

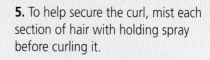

11

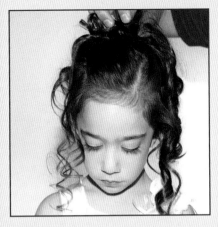

12

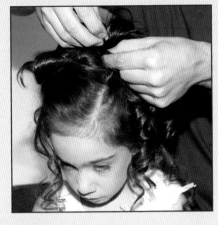

13

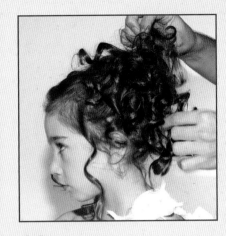

14

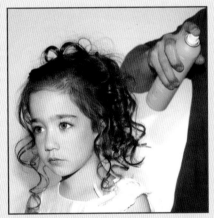

15

12. Be sure to leave a few curls loose around the face as you gather the rest of them into the ponytail. This creates a more graceful look.

13. Using bobby pins, secure the upswept hair all around the ponytail.

14. Draw the hair in the ponytail upwards and pin it so that it hangs in a loose, casual manner all around the ponytail.

15. Mist the hair with holding spray to secure the hairstyle.

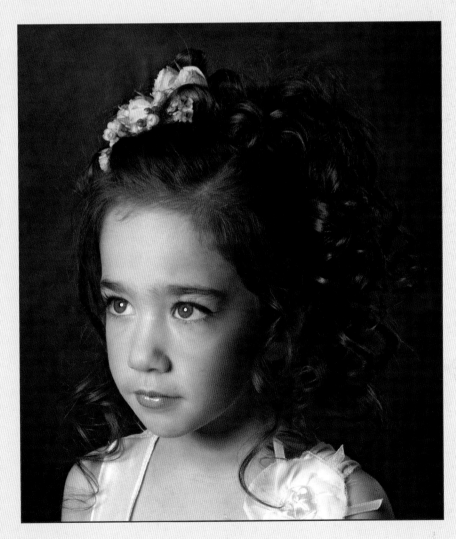

Bridesmaid BEAUTY

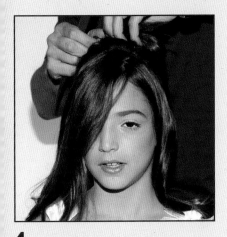

1. Wash and blow dry the hair. Divide the hair into front and back sections by making a part over the crown of the head.

2. Curl the hair that frames the face with a curling iron.

3. Secure each curl with a large clip.

4. Continue to curl all the hair in the front section in this manner.

1

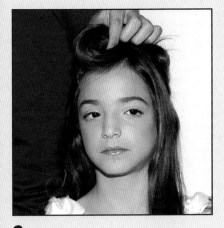

2

This adorable hairstyle easily transforms any young girl into a princess. Sweet and adorable, dress it up with a crescent-shaped flower accessory.

30

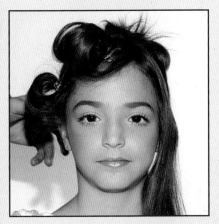

3

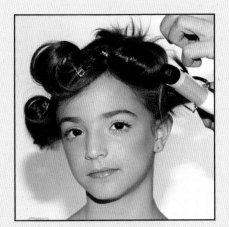

4

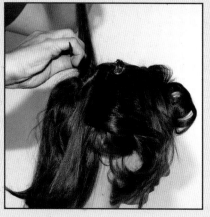

5

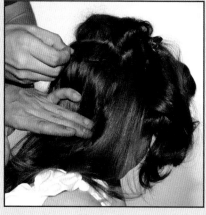

6

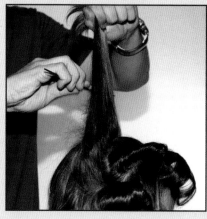

7

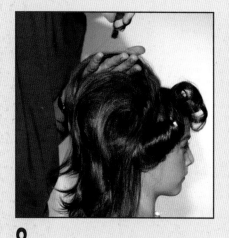

8

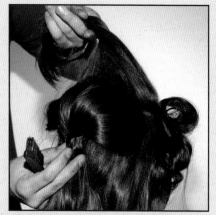

9

5. Grasp a 1-inch wide section of hair at the crown of the head and backcomb it at the roots to add volume. This area will be the base for the hairstyle.

6. Secure the backcombed hair with two bobby pins, inserted to form an X shape.

7. Grasp another 1-inch section of hair and backcomb it at the roots to increase volume.

8. Draw the hair backwards and gently brush the surface for a neat appearance. Mist with a little holding spray.

9. Secure this section of hair at the base of the hairstyle with a few bobby pins.

10. Repeat this technique with another section of hair and pin in at the base with bobby pins. Each of these sections is placed this way to increase volume at the back of the head.

11. Curl the ends of these sections of hair using a curling iron.

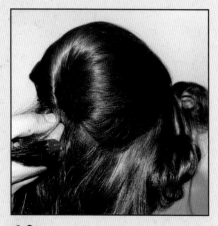

10

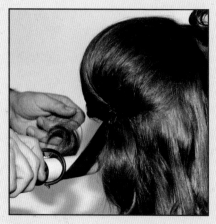

11

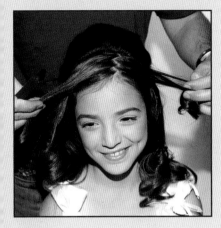
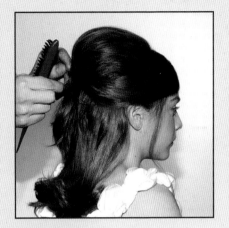
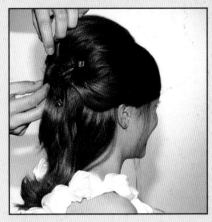

12

13

14

12. Using a tail comb, make a zigzag part in the front section of the hair.

13. Brush the hair from the front towards the back and secure with bobby pins.

14. Roll the ends of this hair into loops and secure with hair clips to create a perfect finish to the hairstyle. Replace the hair clips with bobby pins and mist with hair spray to secure.

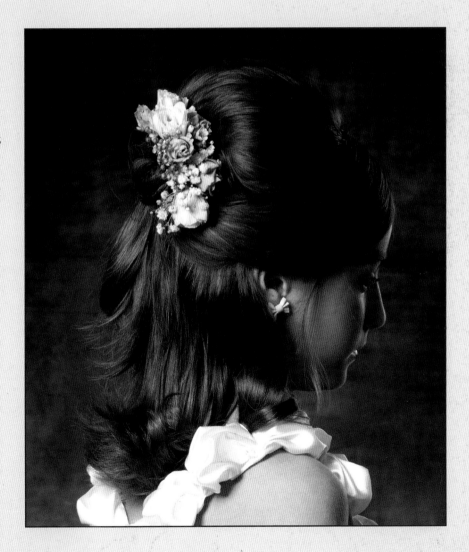

Princess
& PEARLS

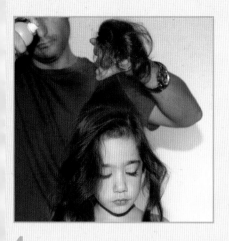

1

1. Wash and blow dry the hair. Mist with holding spray to ensure the style holds better. Divide the hair into front and back sections by making a part over the top of the head and towards the back, from one ear to the other.

2. Gather the hair at the back of the head in a ponytail.

3. Divide the hair at the front of the head into three sections, so that the middle section is above the brow and the other sections are on either side of the face.

4. Draw the sections on the right and left sides of the face towards the back of the head and secure with bobby pins at the base of the ponytail.

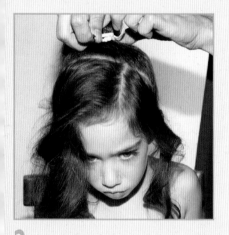

2

For a bridesmaid who wants a touch of sophistication, this hairstyle is a dream come true. Increase the elegance by dressing it up with a strand of pretty pearls.

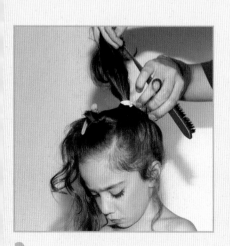

3

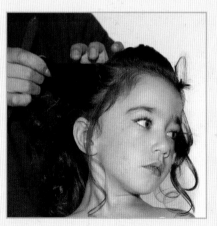

4

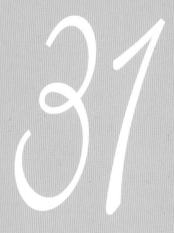

31

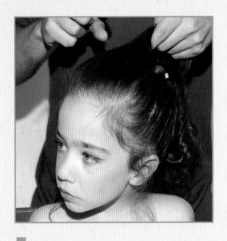

5

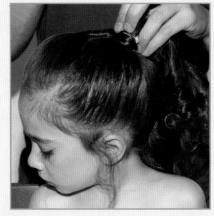

6

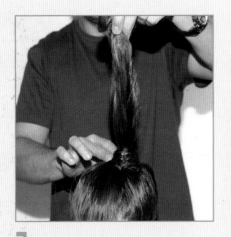

7

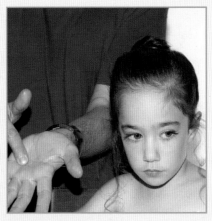

8

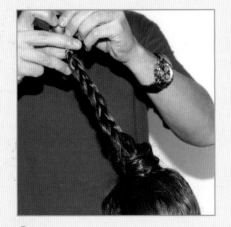

9

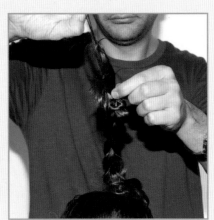

10

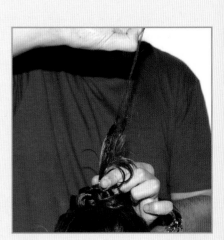

11

5. Mist the hair with holding spray before brushing it backwards.

6. Leave a few strands of hair loose around the face for a softer look.

7. All the hair should now be affixed at one point, at the back of the head in the center.

8. Place a bit of wax on your palms and rub it along the hair in the ponytail.

9. Divide the hair in the ponytail into two sections and braid each section into a loose braid. Secure the end of each braid with an elastic band.

10. Grasp the end of one braid with one hand and push the hair in the braid towards the scalp with the other hand.

11. This technique gives the braid an interesting texture.

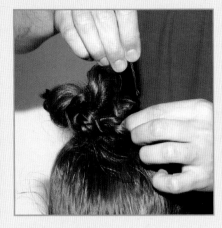

12

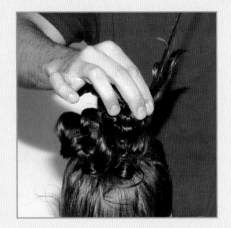

13

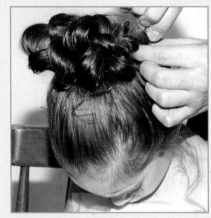

14

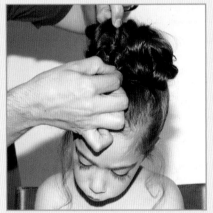

15

12. Wrap the braids around the base of the ponytail and secure with bobby pins.

13. Repeat this technique with the other braid.

14. Position the braids to achieve the desired look and secure with bobby pins.

15. Gently pull strands of hair from both braids to increase the volume of the hairstyle. Mist with holding spray.

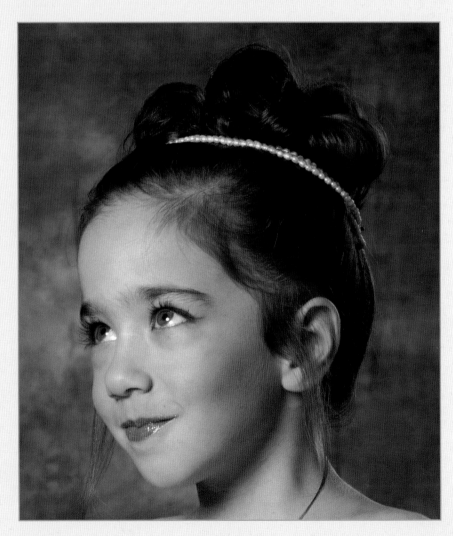

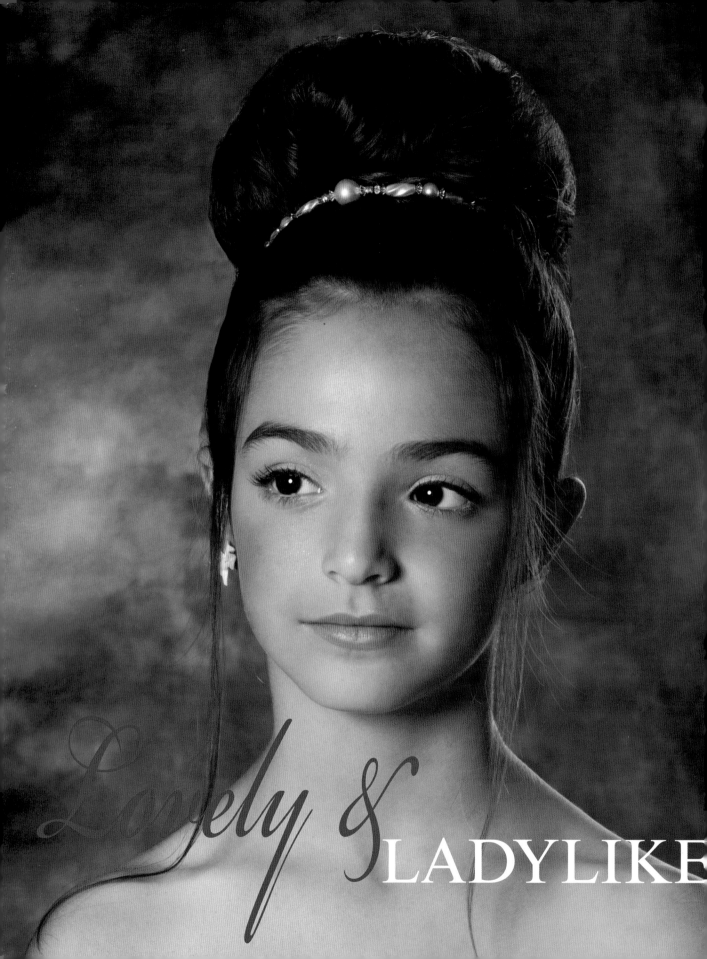

Lovely & LADYLIKE

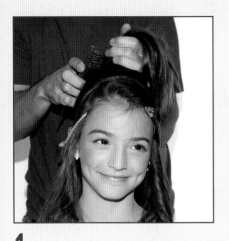

1. Wash and blow dry the hair. Divide the hair into front and back sections by making a part that runs over the crown of the head.

2. Gather a section of hair at the back of the head into a high ponytail.

3. Divide the hair at the front of the head into three sections. Mist the middle section with holding spray.

4. Brush back this section of hair until it is smooth and then draw it towards the ponytail.

1

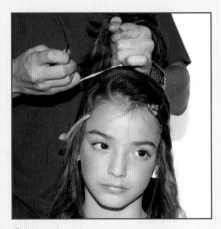

2

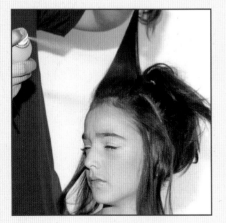

3

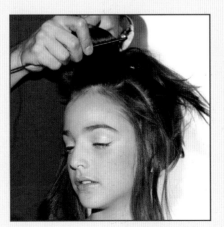

4

This elegant style is ideal for dressing up your teenage bridesmaid. Add a decorative bobby pin or beaded necklace to accessorize with ease.

32

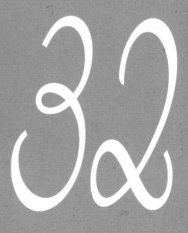

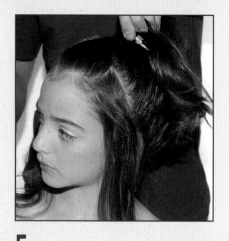

5

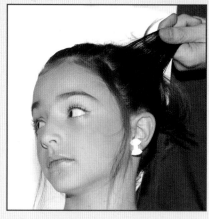

6

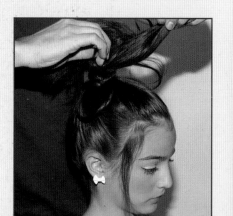

7

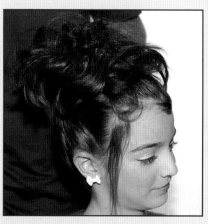

8

5. Secure the hair at the base of the ponytail with bobby pins.

6. Draw back the hair on the left and right sides of the face in the same way, brushing it until it is smooth and pinning it securely near the base of the ponytail. Leave a few strands of hair around the face to create a softer look.

7. Draw the hair in the ponytail upwards and backcomb it at the roots.

8. Backcomb all of the hair in the ponytail for maximum volume.

9. Mist the ponytail with holding spray, at a distance of about 8 inches, to keep the volume.

10. Gently brush the hair on the exterior of the ponytail for a soft look.

11. Brush this part of the ponytail until the ponytail is shaped like a ball and has a smooth exterior. Mist the ponytail with holding spray to secure the shape.

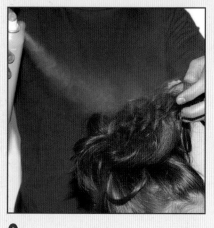

9

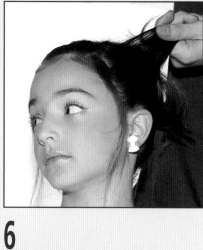

10

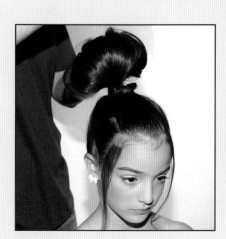

11

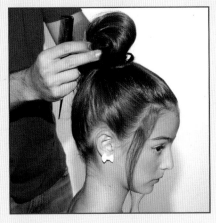

12

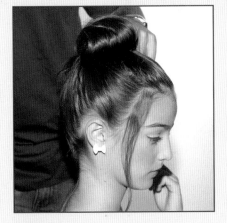

13

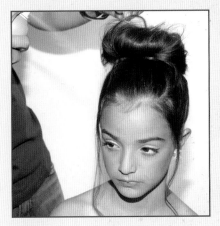

14

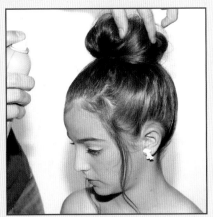

15

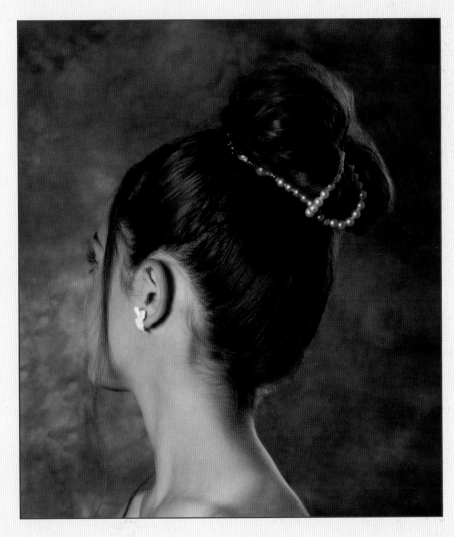

12. With a rolling movement, draw the ends of the hair in the ponytail towards the base of the ponytail.

13. Secure the ends of the ponytail to the scalp with bobby pins. Use more bobby pins to secure the ball-shaped ponytail all around.

14. Mist the entire ponytail with holding spray. Draw out a few strands of hair to give the ball a bit more volume.

15. Mist the entire hairstyle with holding spray to set the look.

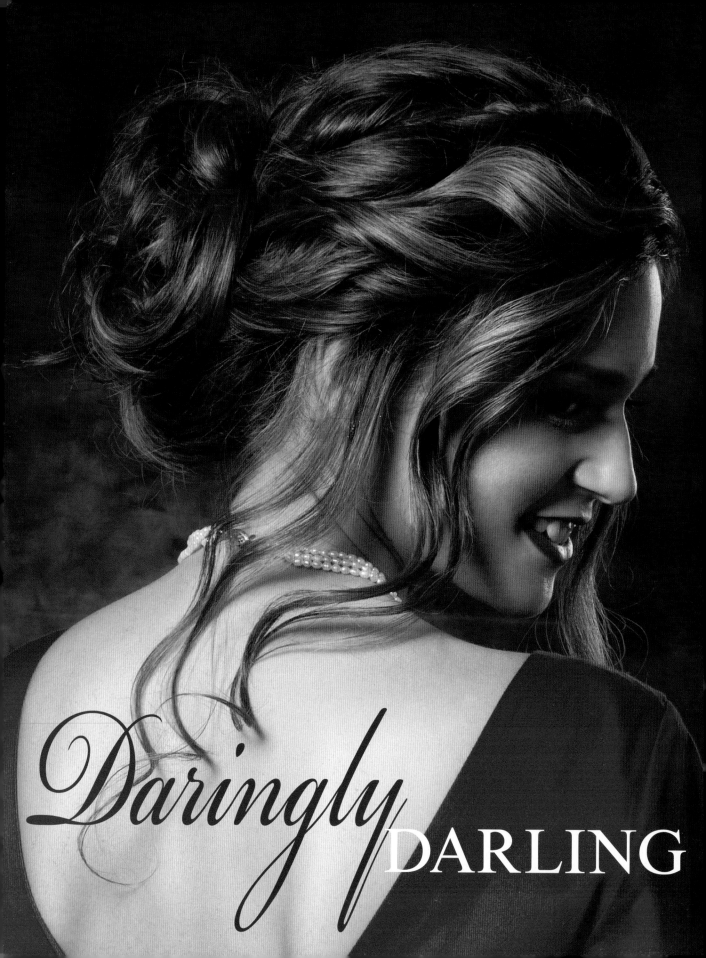

Daringly DARLING

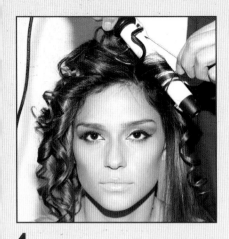

1. Wash and blow dry the hair. Use a curling iron to curl all the hair, one section at a time.

2. Mist the hair with a little holding spray to hold the style for longer.

3. Grasp a section of hair from above each ear and draw the two sections to the back of the head.

4. Secure the sections of hair together at the back of the head with an elastic band. This serves as the base for the hairstyle.

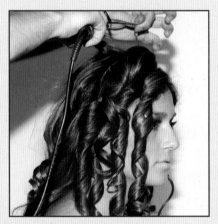

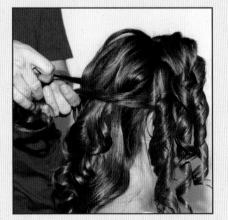

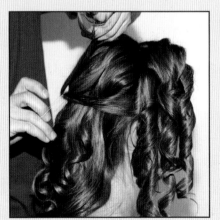

This hairstyle combines an upswept back with a wispy front. It's ideal for any member of the bridal party or for a treasured guest.

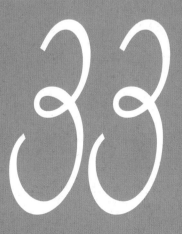

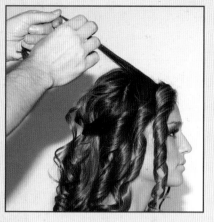

5

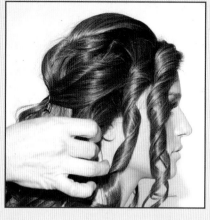

6

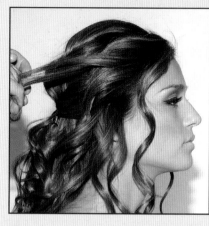

7

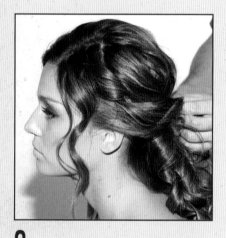

8

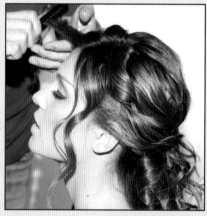

9

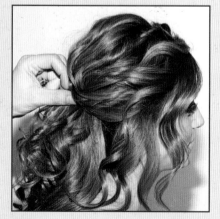

10

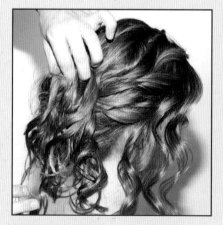

11

5. Gently release the curl in each section of hair, making sure to retain the wave.

6. Pin the waves of hair, section by section, over the base you made in step 4.

7. To create a really romantic look, gather the hair in a gentle, wavy style.

8. When gathering sections of hair from around the face, make sure you allow loose strands of hair to fall freely around the face.

9. To keep the waves open and natural-looking, gently brush each section of curled hair and spray it with a little holding spray.

10. Secure the hair with bobby pins at the base of the hairstyle.

11. Gather about one-third of the hair and roll it upwards, like a rope.

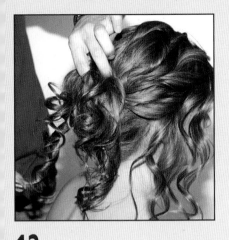

12

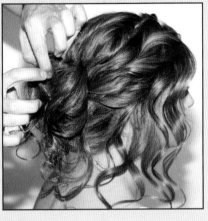

13

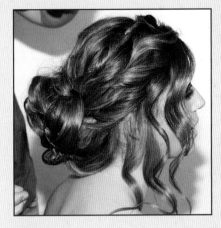

14

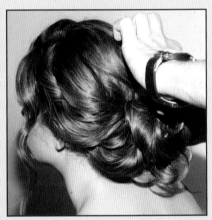

15

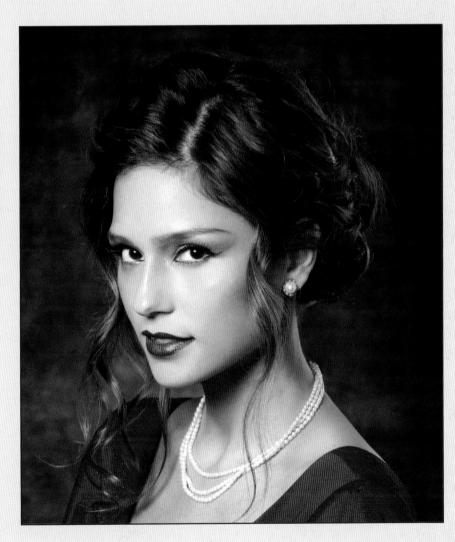

12. Secure the hair to the base of the hairstyle with bobby pins.

13. Gather the remaining two sections of hair in the same way.

14. Continue to gather the remaining loose curls at the back of the head.

15. Mist the entire hairstyle with holding spray to secure it.

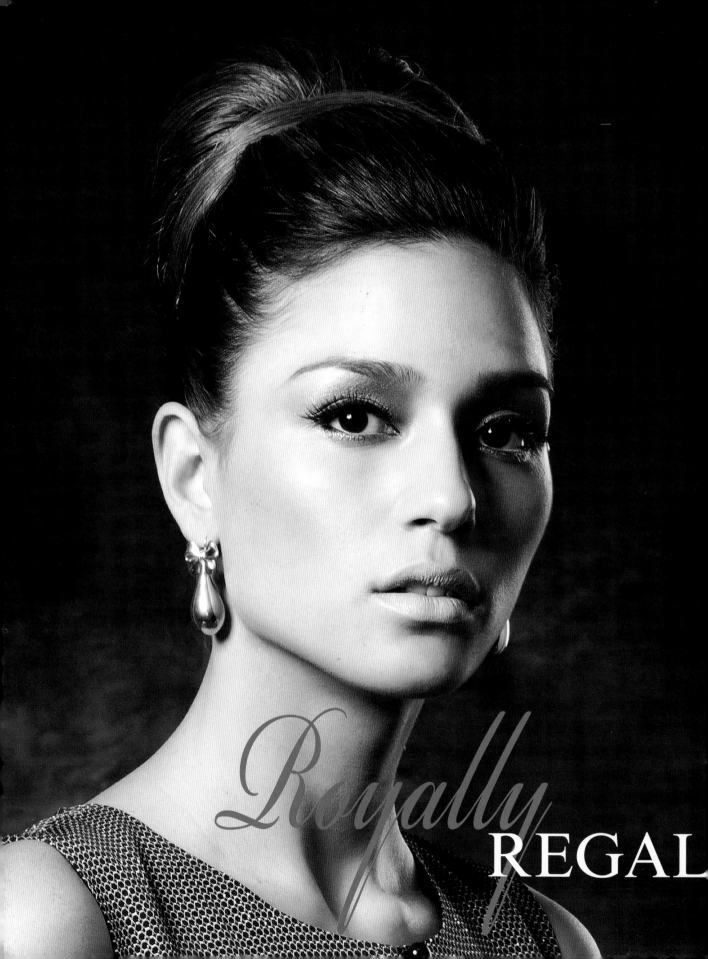

Royally REGAL

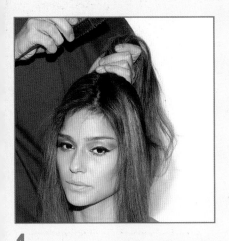

1 **1.** Wash and blow dry the hair. Divide the hair into front and back sections with a part that extends over the crown of the head, from one ear to the other. Gather the hair at the back in a high ponytail.

2. Divide the hair at the front head into three sections: the middle section is above the brow and the other sections are on either side of the face. Draw the sections on the right and left sides of the face towards the base of the ponytail.

3. Grasp a 1-inch section of hair just above the ponytail and backcomb it at the roots to increase volume.

4. Draw this section of hair backwards and gently brush the top of the hair for a smooth, clean look.

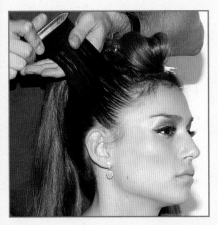

2

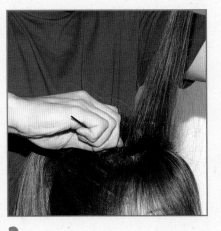

3

4

Radiate elegance and flair with this high oversized bun. With its cleverly concealed hair wrap, it befits a movie star, singer, or mother-of-the-bride.

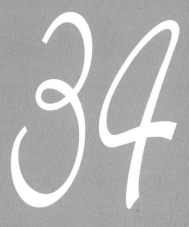

34

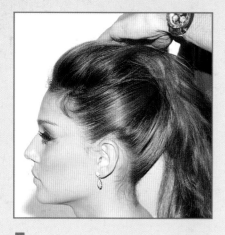

5

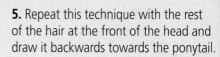
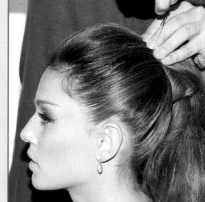

6

5. Repeat this technique with the rest of the hair at the front of the head and draw it backwards towards the ponytail.

6. Insert a bobby pin close to the scalp, aligned with the gathered hair, so that the bobby pin is fastened to one side of the elastic band. Repeat this on the other side, drawing the elastic band on the opposite side and inserting the second pin towards the first one.

7. The elastic band should hold the hair and secure it neatly in place.

8. Divide the hair in the ponytail into three sections: two large sections and one small one. Let the small section hang loose. Pin one of the large sections so that it faces the front of the head. Pin the other large section so that it faces the side.

9. Affix a hair wrap to the base of the ponytail using bobby pins. This wrap will increase the volume of the hairstyle.

10. Brush the hair that was drawn to one side over the hair wrap. Arrange the hair so that it conceals the wrap. Mist with a little holding spray.

11. Tuck in the ends of this section of hair and secure on the opposite side of the hair wrap using bobby pins.

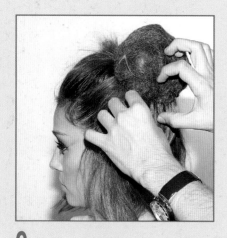

7

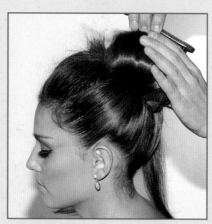

8

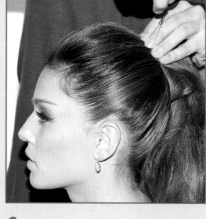

9

10

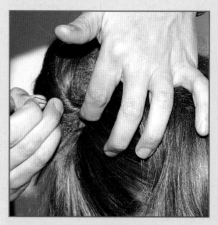

11

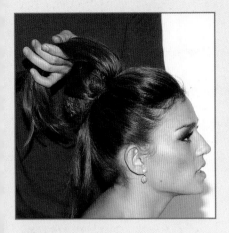

12

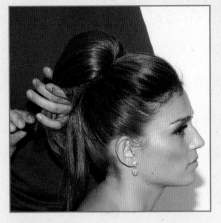

13

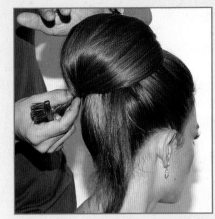

14

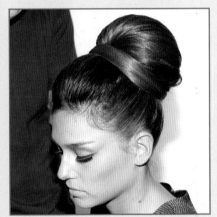

15

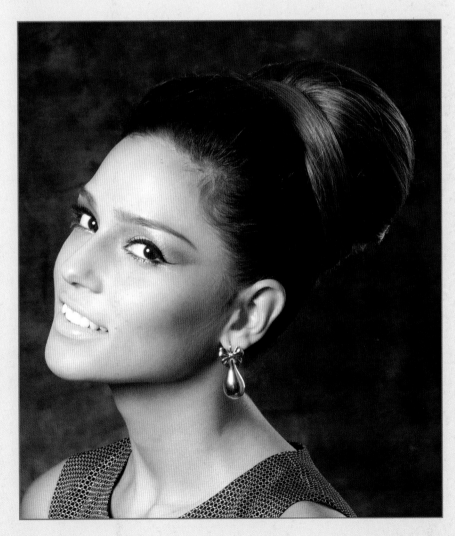

12. Brush the section of hair facing the front of the head backwards and over the hair wrap.

13. Mist this section of hair with holding spray as you brush it backwards in order to create a firmer hold over the hair extension.

14. Draw this hair towards the back of the head and let it curve smoothly under the hair extension. Secure with bobby pins.

15. Wrap the remaining loose section of hair around the front of the large bun you've made with the hair extension and secure with bobby pins. Mist with holding spray.

Index

Acknowledgments

DRESSES

Erez Ovadia
www.erezovadia.com
pages 12, 16, 32, 36, 40, 48, 52, 56, 68, 76, 80, 88, 92, 96, 104

Naama Bezalel
www.naamabezalel.com
pages 8, 20, 24, 28, 60, 64, 84, 108, 116, 136, 140

Ofir Dahan
www.ofir-dahan.co.il
pages 44, 72, 100, 112

Studio Noa
www.studio-noa.co.il
pages 120, 124, 128, 132

EARRINGS

Ayala Vitkon
www.ayala-v.co.il
pages 36, 48, 64, 72, 88, 112

Dama
www.damaline.com
pages 12, 44, 52, 136, 140

Efrat Cassouto
www.efratcassouto.co.il
pages 8, 20, 68, 76, 80, 84, 92, 96, 100, 104, 116

Maor Radijinski
www.maorjd.com
pages 40, 56

Yehezkel Sinai
yehezkel.zah@gmail.com
pages 24, 32

HAIR JEWELRY

Dama
www.damaline.com
pages 28, 44, 111

Efrat Cassouto
www.efratcassouto.co.il
pages 8, 20, 32, 96, 101

Pliskin Creation
www.pliskincreation.com
page 84

Yehezkel Sinai
yehezkel.zah@gmail.com
pages 40, 56, 60

NECKLACES

Ayala Vitkon
www.ayala-v.co.il
pages 12, 28, 72, 88

Dama
www.damaline.com
pages 52, 96, 108

Efrat Cassouto
www.efratcassouto.co.il
pages 16, 48, 68, 92, 104, 116

Pliskin Creation
www.pliskincreation.com
pages 20, 112